MAKE SHI(F)T HAPPEN

Change How You Look by Changing How You Think

Dean Dwyer

Victory Belt Publishing Inc
Las Vegas

To my mom and dad. You gave me the greatest gift of all; the freedom to chose my own direction in life.

Ten percent of the author's royalties will be donated to:

schoolbox.ca

Follow the author at:

beingprimal.com
makeshifthappen.org

First Published in 2012 by Victory Belt Publishing Inc.

ISBN 13: 978-1-936608-70-6

The information included in this book is for educational purposes only. It is not intended nor implied to be a substitute for professional medical advice. The reader should always consult his or her healthcare provider to determine the appropriateness of the information for their own situation or if they have any questions regarding a medical condition or treatment plan. Reading the information in this book does not create a physician-patient relationship.

Victory Belt ® is a registered trademark of Victory Belt Publishing Inc.
Printed in the USA

Table of Contents

Foreword

Typically this section of the book is for the foreword; you know, the section where I get some big name to exaggerate how flippin' awesome I am.

I opted to ditch that section for two reasons. Praise has the same impact on my ego that spring break has on college kids. Both end up going wild and doing or saying something really stupid. More important, this book isn't about me. I wrote it for you so it only makes sense that this space be dedicated to you.

With that, here are 10 things I know to be true about you that you may not know yet.

1. There is a solution to your problem out there, but it's not one of those "one-size-fits-all" things. It's one you will assemble yourself.
2. You are not your genetics. You are what you fight to become.
3. You are the expert on you. NO ONE knows what works for you other than you. NO ONE!
4. Success is a numbers game. All of your past failures tip the percentages in your favor.
5. Someone out there has overcome a situation very similar to yours. That means what you are trying to do is possible.
6. There is a lean, healthy you waiting to be released. You just haven't opened the right door yet.
7. You are merely scratching the surface of your potential.
8. You think you are supposed to solve this problem

yourself. You are not. It's too complex to tackle solo. Surround yourself with people who can help.

9. Belief is contagious. It just needs a starting point. You just gave it one by picking up this book.

10. Regardless of your circumstances, change does not discriminate. It offers its services to anyone that embraces it. Guess what? YOU ARE READY TO EMBRACE IT!

Let's make some shift happen,

Dean

Introduction

REVERSAL
OF
FAILURE

If you are reading this book there are probably three conclusions that I can make with relative certainty. First, you are not happy with the current state of your body. Second, you are looking for a way to create significant change with sustainable results. Third, and most importantly, you recognize that what you are currently doing (or not doing) isn't working. I applaud you for that final insight because change begins by acknowledging that fact.

First of all: it's not your fault! The weight-loss industry has led us astray with the dizzying and contradictory number of fads: eat low-fat, eat high-fat, no carbs are good, no carbs are bad—how can we possibly keep up when diets come and go at a rate that rivals the latest fashion trends? Don't listen to the latest diet guru, listen to your body and, based on what it's telling you, come up with your own plan. I'm not here to be the next expert, but rather to act as your guide through the process of changing how you view weight-loss. I firmly believe based on my own weight-loss experience that you can't change how you look until you make a shift in your thinking about weight-loss.

How do I know? Because I've been where you are and the only way I was able to lose weight was to toss out everything I knew about weight-loss and start at square one, building up my own plan piece-by-piece. I didn't do anything drastic, but rather made a series of small changes that made all the difference in the end.

I have always been frustrated with the fact that many people who claim to be experts at losing weight have never been fat or overweight themselves. They don't really know what we are thinking or understand what is holding us back. Consequently, many of the solutions they provide either don't work or are not sustainable in the long-term.

I get the notion of not wanting to look in a mirror. I get the whole thing about wearing baggy clothes to hide the body that lies underneath. I get that you begin to feel that you just weren't meant to be thin or that you lack the personal fortitude required to make this change a reality.

It's worth repeating again. I GET IT! I have lived all of those feelings. And that's why I can help.

No shirt! No way!

For as long as I can remember, I hated taking my shirt off. I didn't like taking it off at the beach, I didn't like taking it off at home, and I definitely didn't take it off when I was standing in front of a mirror.

I didn't even like taking off my pullovers when I was out in public for fear that my T-shirt underneath would be pulled up as well, exposing my large, ab-less belly to the horrified crowd around me. So I worked hard to ensure my stomach remained hidden from the world.

While I was trying to hide the body I had from others, I was frustrated that no matter how hard I tried I was never able to release the body that I knew was trapped inside.

Take it off!

Eight or nine years ago I was at a buddy's cottage for a guys' week-end. You know what that means! It's a perfect excuse for a bunch of guys to do what guys do best—play cards, drink beer, and generally act like big jackasses.

One day we were playing horseshoes. This "sport" is about as close as you can come to doing nothing aside from actually doing noth-ing. But it provides a great opportunity for trash talking among a bunch of washed-up, aging, former high school "superstars."

It was a blazing hot day, and while I was only wearing a T-shirt and shorts, I was still sweating profusely. The solution was simple—take my shirt off, but I was reluctant to do so.

It's weird how I can still remember the emotional struggle of that de-cision. My internal dialogue must have gone on for fifteen or twenty minutes. Finally, I thought to myself, "Dude, I'm with a bunch of guys. I could cut my arm off and throw that instead of the horseshoe and these bozos wouldn't even notice."

So I took my shirt off. And you know what? I could not have been more wrong. They noticed.

After doing a quick double take, one of my friends shot a glance down at my protruding white belly and quipped, "Whoa! That's a lot of carrots!" in reference to my decade-long vegetarian diet. It was a great line, even if it was at my own expense, but more importantly, it was the moment I first realized my vegetarian diet wasn't doing anything for my physique.

Twenty-five years of doing the wrong thing...

When I look back, my struggle with weight gain actually started in college. Those years were lean when it came to money, studying, and decent grades, but not so lean when it came to my ability to store body fat.

Even though I had started working out and watching what I ate, by the time I got to the final year of my undergraduate degree, my five-foot nine-inch frame had soared up to 215 pounds (the heaviest I have ever been and about 50 pounds above my ideal weight).

The twenty-five years that followed were spent chasing this vision of my ideal physique: I worked out like a dog (well, not like a real dog, although if you throw a tennis ball I will run and chase it), was vegetarian/vegan, and seldom ate fast food or junk food.

And yet I was still overweight.

In November 2010, after twenty-five years of failure, I reached a boiling point. The struggle with my weight had led to nothing but immense frustration. I was tired of having nothing to show for my efforts. I was also fed up with the weight-loss industry as a whole. It did not make the path to weight-loss clearer, but instead cluttered it with swaths of contradictory and misinformed ideas.

The largest part of my frustration was directed at myself. Try as I might, I could never get rid of the big, disgusting roll of fat around my midsection.

Sure there were times when I seemed to make some progress but, for reasons I could never fully comprehend, I always managed to find my way back to a less-than-ideal weight.

My brewing frustration led to an "epiphany." I use quotation marks because I was no stranger to epiphanies. I had one every six months or so, and after each one I always thought, "This is it! My life will never be the same." And it wasn't . . . for a while. But I would always find a way to resort back to my old fat self. Needless to say, I was a tad leery of this latest one.

There was no reason for me to believe that this time would be different, and yet I couldn't shake the feeling that I was onto something this time because my epiphany focused not on how to lose weight, but rather on how to think about weight-loss. Twenty-five years of doing "stuff" hadn't worked. This time I needed to be different, and in order for me to be different, I needed to think differently.

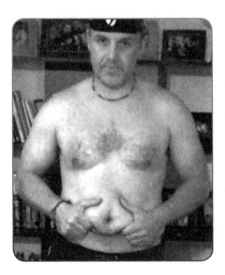 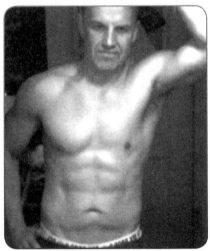

Finding ideas everywhere...

Through lots of reading, research, self-experimentation, and thought, I came up with twenty shifts. Each shift led to a subtle change in thinking that in turn allowed the subsequent shift to come more easily, until the accumulation of shifts resulted in a complete mental overhaul. The results were both successful and sustainable, without the melodrama of forcing a single drastic change that I couldn't keep up over the long-term.

Can this series of shifts work for you?

Why not? There is nothing magical about what I did. You just need to begin to embrace BEING DIFFERENT and commit to adding new, manageable behaviors that allow for transformation to happen. Once that occurs, then shift can't help but follow.

DO SOMETHING SEISMIC ⇨

Around the time that I decided I needed to do things differently, I picked up *The Dragonfly Effect* by Jennifer Aaker and Andy Smith, and one of the phrases I came across while skimming the introduction by Chip Heath was this:

DO SOMETHING SEISMIC!

While Heath was referring to the art of social media, I was nonetheless completely captivated by those three words and knew that I needed to apply them to my quest to transform my body. After decades of dormant thinking, I was desperate to invite a little seismic activity into my life.

The simple premise of *The Dragonfly Effect* is:

Small actions can create enormous change.

I loved this idea for the mere fact that I always thought it was the other way around, that big change was caused by monstrous action. The bigger the problem, the bigger the action I attempted to take.

The problem with this go-big-or-go-home attitude is that it is impossible to sustain over time. Sure, we can force our bodies to do some unreasonable things for a short duration, but at some point, most are so unreasonable for our particular set of circumstances that they simply become unsustainable.

BULLSHI(F)T: *More is better*

Back in the late 1990s I decided that I would work out twice a day. If I worked out more often, I would increase my fitness, right? I started doing forty-five minutes of mind-numbingly, boring cardio in the morning and forty-five minutes of repetitive resistance training in the evening.

Needless to say, my short-lived experiment in working out twice a day was not a success. Maybe if I had been unemployed with no relationship or social life to speak of I could have pulled it off, but it was just not a sustainable strategy long-term.

THE RIGHT SHI(F)T: *Better is better*

Whatever you decide to do must add value while also being sustainable over time. Do something that fits into the context of who you are and how you live your life. Don't force something that doesn't mesh with your lifestyle or philosophy—it won't last.

The first step...

After my November 2010 realization that I had to be and think differently, I knew that I needed to do something **SEISMIC**. I accomplished this by thinking small rather than big and attempting to perform a series of seemingly insignificant actions that could have a dramatic impact on what my body would look like.

While I had no idea how well these things would play out, I ended up isolating nineteen other strategies in an attempt to create something I had never achieved before . . . a LEAN body.

How to think seismically...

You might be wondering how to actually implement the "going seismic" philosophy. The first thing I did to get the ball rolling was to stop thinking about my struggle within the narrow focus of weight-loss. I had to zoom out the lens in order to see that it was not about losing weight, it was about understanding how to rid myself of unwanted behaviors and adopting new ones that would make weight-loss possible.

So I rejected any and all things that focused solely on outcome. In other words, I didn't give a rat's ass about the scale and how much I weighed.

Instead I reasoned that if I adopted the right behaviors, the weight-loss would eventually follow.

Finding the right behaviors for you...

I'm a huge nonfiction reader. One of the books I was reading during my attempted transition from fat to lean was *Influencer: The Power to Change Anything*.

The book mentions that the National Weight Control Registry (a registry I didn't even know existed) had statistics on the three vital behaviors utilized by people who lost at least thirty pounds and had kept it off for a minimum of six years.

1. They worked out from home

2. They ate breakfast

3. They weighed themselves daily

I personally don't endorse the third behavior, but the first one really intrigued me because I never thought I could work out from home.

But it had become apparent over the past few years that I could not work out at the gym either. I had morphed into that guy who was now donating a monthly fee to NOT go.

As I started to think about working out at home, I began to see how it could be extremely beneficial to adopt this behavior.

Why gyms don't work for most people...

While a gym certainly works for some, for most there is a huge barrier in just getting to the gym. Just think of all the steps it takes:

⇨ You have to psych yourself up just to get your butt out of the house.

⇨ You have to pack like you are going on a sleepover.

⇨ You need to drive to the destination and most likely battle some kind of traffic.

⇨ You need to find and often pay for parking—or the parking ticket you get when you underestimate how long your workout will take.

⇨ You need to figure out what kind of a workout you want to do and battle for equipment usage.

⇨ If you are taking any popular classes, you need to arrive early just to ensure you get on the list.

⇨ And then you need to factor in the time it takes to get back home.

All these variables conspire to keep you from going to the gym.

So as I began to break this down, I realized working out from home only required that I psych myself up. I could not only cut out the other potential obstacles, but I could also gain some positives:

⇨ No packing/unpacking, wardrobe change, or lugging a gym bag required.

⇨ I could do my workouts on my own time schedule.

⇨ I saved at least 60 minutes because I didn't have to drive, circle around looking for a parking spot, arrive early to reserve spots for classes, and so on.

⇨ I pocketed at least $600/year on membership fees (or as I see it; I gained one return ticket to Vancouver to visit my brother).

⇨ By keeping the car parked, I saved on gas, parking, and potential insurance hikes by reducing my risk of being in an accident.

⇨ I didn't have to worry about some hairy, naked dude bending over in front of me to put on his socks before his underwear. *Seriously guys, what's up with that?*

Little did I know just how seismic that small behavior change would be in my overall transformation!

MAKE SHI(F)T HAPPEN...

1 Consider doing some (if not all) of your workouts from home. Before you explain why you can't work out from home, keep in mind that I used to have the same excuses. You can learn to work out from home. I'm proof of that.

CREATING CHANGE IS NOTHING OTHER THAN TEACHING YOURSELF NEW BEHAVIORS!

2 Train yourself to start thinking that small, seemingly inconsequential actions can create seismic change if you can commit to repeating them over time. The mere act of logging everything I ate each day was a major reason I have been able to achieve what I have achieved. I expand on that more in Shift #16: Log like Captain Kirk.

THINK BIG! BUT ACT SMALL!

3 There are all kinds of great and useful pieces of equipment that you can purchase at reasonable prices that will allow you to create an amazing workout for yourself at home. Here are a few that I personally use and LOVE . . .

The Ultimate Body Press (all in one dip station)
www.ultimatebodypress.com

Ultimate Sandbag Core Training System
www.ultimatesandbagtraining.com

Studbar Pull-up Bar
www.studbarpullup.com

To learn more about this and other innovative solutions to creating your own home gym head over to

www.makeshifthappen.org/resources

TRAIN YOURSELF TO WORK OUT FROM HOME AND REMOVE THE BARRIERS THAT PREVENT MANY PEOPLE FROM SUCCEEDING!

IGNORE MOST (BUT NOT ALL) EXPERTS ⇨

Now that I had boarded the Do Something Seismic Express, I began to think about other ways I could change my outlook. Looking over my body of work (pun intended) from the previous twenty-five years of failure, I realized I always defaulted to the same behavior when I gained weight. Instead of really figuring out the root cause of my weight gain, I merely tried different weight-loss strategies on for size, hoping something would fit. This way I could feel like I was being proactive. Even if what I was doing wasn't working, I was at least trying, right?

Time to tee it up...

If we keep our eyes and ears open, inspiration can come from the most unlikely of sources.

In my case, it actually came from something that Tiger Woods once said in an interview where he attributed part of his success (I'm referring to his golf game of course, not his ability to juggle multiple sexual partners) to his ability to "think his way around the golf course."

I loved this because it implied that golf was not simply about hitting a little white ball into a hole in the ground. It was far more complex and intricate. It had nuances and subtleties that required a much deeper understanding of the course, the game, and one's own abilities.

It dawned on me that I was not thinking my way around the tricky terrain that was my body and the things I could be doing to enhance its transformation.

To the contrary, I was outsourcing my thinking to the so-called experts, who couldn't possibly know my body or my specific set of circumstances.

Experts had gotten me nowhere . . .

It became apparent that there was a serious bug in the Dean Dwyer operating system.

Each time I wanted to create massive change in my life, I would assume that some expert out there had the solution. But relying on experts was actually part of my problem.

It's not that they aren't trying to be helpful; it's just that most (not all) make the same fundamental mistakes.

First, they falsely believe that if everyone does exactly what they do, then everyone will achieve exactly what they have achieved.

Each body is as unique as the fingerprints that accompany it, so the "one-size-fits-all" mentality is strategically flawed thinking that just doesn't work for most people.

BULLSHI(F)T: *"Lose 20 pounds in 30 days"*

This is an actual ad that I have seen on a number of websites. Unless the plan requires surgical removal of a body part or two, there is no way that any company can or should be making such a claim.

Sadly, these ads are everywhere and extremely effective with those desperate to lose weight quickly. But if you were to critically assess this advertisement, you would note two things immediately.

First, it is focuses solely on outcomes. There is absolutely no talk of behavior change, so it's logical to assume that any "forced" losses would not be sustainable over time.

Second, it makes the assumption that weight-loss is linear. Interest earned on $5,000 in a month is linear. Weight-loss is like the stock market. It's volatile and unpredictable.

THE RIGHT SHI(F)T: *Adopt twenty shifts!*

Do not attach body transformation goals that are measured in units of time or pounds. Instead, commit to acquiring and maintaining high-leverage behaviors that lead to stellar results. (Psst! I know twenty shifts you can adopt.)

Second, they think we all react exactly the same to any particular stimulus.

Just because something works for you does not mean it will work for me. The problem is many of us have been conditioned to think that if it worked for someone else, then it MUST work for us as well.

If we blindly buy into the idea that everyone responds to stimuli in a similar fashion, then when it doesn't work, we either think we are the problem because our body doesn't respond correctly or we think we are the problem because we must be doing something wrong. The natural assumption that follows is to believe we are defective or lack the character required to achieve what everyone else seems to be achieving.

Third, many experts don't really understand their own success.

I have listened to far too many who attribute their successes to factors and clichés that didn't really have anything to do with their success.

One of the most glaring I hear is, "You have to work hard." Seriously, what does that even mean? It's one of the most useless pieces of advice out there, and a great indicator of someone who has no clue why they succeeded in the first place.

Why is it useless? It lacks guidance. It lacks direction. It lacks insight. There is absolutely nothing that someone can do with that piece of information. It's the art of saying something without actually saying anything at all.

For those playing along at home, it's not about working harder; it's about working better by leveraging behaviors that get stellar results. And how do you do that? Not by blindly following the experts, but by starting with an idea and meticulously testing your own theories to find out what works for your body type.

Fourth, they omit the details.

I attended an Anthony Robbins seminar, and let me tell you, this guy is a master of motivation. Seriously, I wanted to run home afterward. I thought better of it when I realized I had actually flown to the conference.

One of the stories he shared was being this eighteen-year-old kid living in a 400-square-foot apartment, doing his dishes in the bathtub and being completely broke. Within a year he managed to completely turn his life around and become a millionaire.

The story was incredibly inspiring, but I was never able to do anything with it to create change in my own life. Now I know why. He didn't give me any details that I could actually act upon.

I needed to know what happened on Day 1. What actions did he take? What was he thinking? What behaviors did he adopt? Did he bathe and do his dishes at the same time?

If a chef won't reveal his secret ingredient, will you be able to replicate his star dish?

Details help us connect the dots in our own lives. When experts omit these, they omit the possibility that others can also reach the same results in their own lives.

Fifth, some have a hidden agenda.

Many experts are simply out to sell you their products and services. Now there is nothing wrong with this, because that is how these people (myself included) make their living.

But there is a way to do this without using sly techniques to manipulate people. It drives me bananas when people use psychology to manipulate others into buying stuff they probably don't need.

BULLSHI(F)T: *The product is principal*

Bill Phillips wrote *Body for Life* back in 1999. I bought it and quite liked it. It served its purpose for me at the time, but one of the things I found disturbing was that every daily meal plan listed in the book included at least two of his meal replacement products.

This is the problem I had and still have with people who do this. Are you committed to my success, or are you using the book as a way to simply sell your product? *Note: supplements have a MUCH higher profit margin than books do.*

There are plenty of ways to do this ethically of course. I follow Chris Guillebeau at www.chrisguillebeau.com. He blogs about work, life, and travel. He has an ever-expanding array of products on offer, but always makes it clear that they are just options and those interested in coming for the free advice and leaving the buying to others will have plenty to choose from.

THE RIGHT SHI(F)T: *The Principle is the Product*

Select mentors based on those who promote principles rather than products. They are more apt to give you balanced, unbiased advice.

Sixth, they make you dependent upon their services.

Experts should help you build behaviors that would eventually put them out of a job. Yes, you read that correctly. Experts are either helping you develop behaviors that allow you to fly solo or they are pushing just enough advice so that you have to keep returning to the nest. If experts are truly committed to helping you, they should want to set you free, not cage you in.

If their intent is dependency, cut them loose.

MAKE SHI(F)T HAPPEN...

1 Not all experts are created equal. We need to carefully evaluate them before blindly buying into what they have to offer. Here are some tips on how to become an expert spotter of experts:

✓ They are incredibly transparent in all that they do.

✓ They don't manipulate with psychology.

✓ They encourage you to seek out and try other options.

✓ They are open about their flaws and struggles.

✓ They don't claim to have all the answers.

✓ They are brutally honest.

✓ They emphasize the process rather than the outcome.

✓ They don't make you commit to some ridiculous long-term contract.

CHOOSE EXPERTS CAREFULLY!

---

2 Even after you've decided a particular expert is worth your time and energy, don't take everything he or she says without question. It is still your job to be your own curator and figure out what information should be applied to your specific circumstances.

Test everything on yourself and draw your own conclusions. Nothing is fact until you have gathered your own empirical data. Ideas are then accepted or rejected based on how they work for you and your particular body type.

BECOME THE EXPERT ON YOU!

3 A good example of an expert with the right attitude is the paleo diet expert Robb Wolf. He doesn't take himself too seriously, and his humor is often at his own expense. Also, while he believes whole-heartedly in the Paleolithic lifestyle, he is not going to force it down your throat. On the contrary, he encourages people to try a variety of dietary lifestyles and decide what works best for them.

If you are interested in adding him to your inner circle of select experts and would like to learn more about Robb, go to www.robbwolf.com.

He also wrote the *New York Times* bestseller, *The Paleo Solution*, which is a great primer on living the ancestral lifestyle.

CHANGE YOUR MIND ⇨

The mind is a funny thing. It can be our greatest resource or our worst enemy. Left to its own devices it can become a toxic breeding ground for thoughts that seek to crush your dreams, undermine your desires, cast large shadows of doubt on your abilities, and prey on your insecurities.

As I ventured into season twenty-five of Operation Fat Loss, I knew that I had to declutter all the negative thoughts hoarded in my mind if I was going to make room for new ideas.

The real question was how to clean house without falling back on some of the lame-o tactics I had used in the past.

Death to clichés...

Aspirational mumbo jumbo and clichés won't create change: it's too unspecific and will quickly be shelved next to other useless trivia. I mean, seriously, if someone told you to be the change you want to see in the world, wouldn't you want to drop kick him right in his Gandhi-like ass?

Don't get me wrong. I love the thought. And I get it intellectually, but what I am supposed to takeaway from it? The concept is so immense there isn't really an applicable starting point.

But a starting point is exactly what you need if you are going to have any success with changing your thoughts. Something Malcolm Gladwell wrote in *The Tipping Point* comes to mind.

Applying the Broken Windows Theory...

Malcolm Gladwell actually exposed me to two mind-blowing ideas in his book *The Tipping Point*.

The first was discovering that I was not the only one who suffered from a rare hair follicle mutation called Big Hairitis. It afflicts 1 out of every 3 billion people.

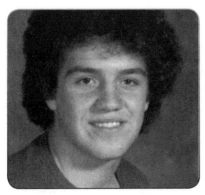

[That is me and my fro circa 1983. Is it just me or does the word "MEOW" come to mind.]

Second, he introduced me to the Broken Windows Theory.

The theory was based on a study done by criminologists James Wilson and George Kelling who noted that normal law abiding citizens were more likely to partake in unlawful behavior (i.e., throw a rock through the window of an abandoned building) if a window was already broken.

The theory implies that the broken window acts as a stimulus for unlawful behavior because it sends a message that no one cares. And if people get the slightest whiff of "anything goes," anarchy is not far behind.

Let's take an example of something that is quite common in a big city: graffiti. While it may seem trivial, graffiti sends a message to potential criminals that no one is going to take action. They target such areas because they reason that their chances of getting caught are greatly reduced. This in turn invites more daring crimes like muggings and robberies, and these become a precursor to more violent crime.

The solution? Remove the initial stimulus and you remove the likelihood of unlawful behavior.

As Gladwell states,
> "An epidemic [crime in this case] can be reversed ... by tinkering with the tiniest details of the immediate environment."

The theory is brilliant, and the implications are *immense* because it smashes the idea that we should not sweat the small stuff. We have to sweat the small stuff because it is the small stuff that eventually escalates into *big* stuff.

What I love even more is that the principle can be used across multiple disciplines where behavior change is required. Parents can use it, teachers can use it, and police departments can use it.

The New York City Police Department used it to reduce a skyrocketing crime rate back in the 1990s by focusing on the precursors to major crime: graffiti, subway fare jumping, aggressive panhandling, public drunkenness, and other such minor offenses.

For instance, if a subway car was vandalized with graffiti, it was immediately taken off the track and repainted. The key was to address these seemingly smaller irrelevant acts of crime immediately and send a very public message that someone was watching.

The results: New York became the safest big city in the country by the end of the 1990s.

MINDSET SHIFT: *Think like a tinker*

I adopted the Broken Windows Theory when I was a teacher and wanted to reduce behavioral issues among my students. With the help of Jim Greene, I pinpointed social skills as a precursor to improved behaviors. In Gladwell's terms, if "behavioral issues" was the epidemic I wanted to reverse, "social skills" were the tiny details that needed tinkering with.

So I tinkered. I didn't just explain that the kids needed to get along; together we broke down, modeled, and practiced the skills required to get along. I didn't just tell them they needed to listen; we dissected what listening looked and sounded like, modeled, and practiced. "Getting along" and "listening" were no longer empty phrases to the kids. They knew what they meant and as a result their behavioral issues decreased.

THE RIGHT SHI(F)T: *Tinker like a tinker*

No one has a "talent" for body transformation: the skills necessary to transform your body are learned. If you are constantly tinkering with your skills, improving them, making them better, then a body transformation will follow. Take willpower. Most people agree that you need it to make changes to your body, but they speak about willpower as an object that one either does or doesn't have in their possession. It didn't get lost in the mail, you didn't miss the two-for-one sale on willpower at the mall. You develop willpower from scratch. It's a learned behavior.

For more on boosting the willpower skill, take a look at *Switch* by Chip and Dan Heath.

Going from theory to practice . . .

We get bombarded with thousands of negative thoughts and images each and every day. If we apply the Broken Windows Theory, then it is logical to assume that if these thoughts are left unattended they will attract more of the same.

In my case I knew if I didn't get in there and clean up the environment, I was going to have a bunch of thoughts behaving like teenagers on spring break. But instead of *Girls Gone Wild*, I was going to be dealing with "thoughts gone wild."

Throwing out everything at once was too daunting, so I focused on the details.

First, I stopped reading the newspaper and watching the news.

The news is set up to do one thing: scare the crap out of us by focusing on all the negative stuff going on in the world. I didn't want all that negativity cluttering my mind, so I stopped watching and reading sensationalist news.

Second, I stopped defending my dietary choices.

Constantly making excuses would only plant doubt and confusion in my mind and attract more of the same, so I stopped defending my nutritional choices. Not only did it clear my thinking, it had the great side effect of reducing the amount of effort and energy I wasted on intricate defense mechanisms.

Third, I developed a strategy to replace negative thoughts with positive ones.

I knew that making catchall comments like "I need to think positive" wasn't going to cut it for me. Anything that was too vague and or focused solely on outcome would just clutter my mind with useless clichés, which was basically another form of negativity.

Since I'm a visual learner, I also knew that more concrete ideas weren't going to sink in by mere recitation. I am a complete idiot when it comes to oral directions. I understand the words, but translating them into actions that actually get me where I want to go seldom works. I always arrive someplace. It's just that the majority of the time it is the wrong place.

So I worried that perhaps my mind would do the same thing with this journey . . . you know, take me to a place I didn't want to go.

When I presented my dilemma to my mom, she suggested that I create a visual representation of the positive things I wanted to focus on.

So instead of just relying on quotes or advice that would quickly be forgotten, I actually took my mom's advice and created the smallest book in the world titled . . .

"How to be Great at My Life."

I took a three-by-five recipe card and folded it in half. The cover contained the title. Inside I handwrote all of the elements that I felt would make my life GREAT.

It currently has over twenty statements of things I would like to achieve in order to be great at my life, ranging from:

✓ *Making kindness my default reaction (replacing my current default reaction: karate chopping people in the carotid artery)*

✓ *Earning an income entirely on products I create*

✓ *Leaving a lasting legacy*

✓ *Extending my influence by becoming a published author (if you are reading this then I can check that bad boy off!)*

✓ *Participating in a school building project (www.schoolbox.ca)*

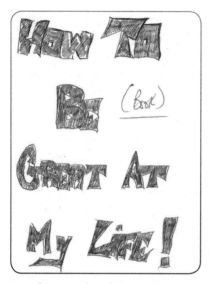

Only a few of my statements revolve solely on my physical appearance because if we focus on changing behaviors, body transformation will naturally follow. Plus, our body is merely a vehicle for all the great things we want to do with our lives.

After I made my book, I would read my list daily to stay focused on what was truly important to me. I would also read them out loud whenever possible, so I could actually hear myself saying the words. The combination of the visual representation and my recitation really worked.

I know it sounds goofy, but the simple notion of replacing negative thoughts with positive ones works because over time you begin to habitually make the positive thoughts your default thoughts.

As an added bonus, if you believe in the Law of Attraction, then you also begin to notice that positive thoughts attract more positive thoughts, which is never a bad thing.

MAKE SHI(F)T HAPPEN...

1 Why not give this a shot and create your own book. Seriously, it costs nothing but your time. It will be just like arts and craft time back when you were in kindergarten, minus the obligatory class clown who used to eat all the glue.

1. Get one three-by-five recipe card (or recycle one of those lame-ass company Christmas cards you got last year).

2. Create a title. Feel free to steal mine.

3. Brainstorm a list of great things you want to have happen in your life.

4. Organize them into different roles or groups. For instance, you could have a section for body transformation, family, work, community, etc.

5. Handwrite them to make this really authentic. (Note: If you are a Doctor DO NOT handwrite these because you will have no clue what you wrote. Get your assistant to do this.)

BE GREAT AT YOUR LIFE!

2 For the technologically savvy, use a free program like Audacity to record an MP3 that you can listen to while in your car, on a walk, or on a break at work. If you are a Mac user, Garage Band is perfect for this.

BE YOUR VOICE OF REASON & INSPIRATION!

3 Do yourself a favor and pick up a copy of any of Malcolm Gladwell's books, whether it is *The Tipping Point*, *Blink*, or *Outliers*. Just remember to read these with the idea of appropriating principles that you can apply to your own personal journey.

To learn more about Gladwell, head to his personal site at www.gladwell.com

TIP LIFE IN YOUR FAVOR!

Shift #17

THINK
IN BETA ⇨

I am the type of perfectionist who procrastinates. If I can't do something perfectly, I'll postpone things until I can get it exactly right. There are pros and cons to this genetic peccadillo, but the cons tend to overshadow the pros because they keep me from doing some of the riskier (yet more rewarding) things in my life.

To counter my perfectionist-caused procrastination, I have unsuccessfully tried to motivate myself with quotes and clichés, as mentioned in the last shift. But I already had enough experience to know that would get me nowhere (I even once tried to apply the Nike slogan "Just Do It" to my life to futile results because the phrase is so outcome-based I had no idea how to Just Do It).

If I was going to succeed at body transformation this time around, I needed to find a way to reframe it.

A "HOLY SHI(F)T" moment...

"IT" hit me while I was reading the book *Rework* by the guys at 37 Signals.

Their brilliant book is littered with insights that are applicable not only to business, but to all areas of your life. I got to thinking about how all of their insights evolved through their efforts to build great software. If I wanted to change my body this time around, I needed to recode the very structure of my thought process.

I needed to think like a software developer.

Here is what I like about software developers that get *it*. They come up with an idea for an application and set about *quickly* designing it until they have a model that is functional. Notice I said functional, *not perfect*. They then release a *beta* version for the world to try out.

What I love about the word *beta* is that it implies the system isn't perfect. It implies there are bugs that will need to be ironed out and features that will need to be updated, added, or removed altogether. And when those updates happen, version 2.0 is born.

The whole process then starts all over again with each new version improving on the previous. And the brilliance of all this is that the improvement never stops. There will always be updates to a newer version.

That is precisely how I have chosen to look at the reshaping of my body. In the past, when the beta version had bugs, I ditched the entire program. That's crazy. That would be the equivalent of Jack Dorsey ditching Twitter simply because of a software glitch (and he had many).

What I needed to remember was that I wasn't going to get it right on version 1.0. Hell, not even on version 2.0. Some of my theories were going to be wrong, some of my exercises were going to suck, and some of my meals were going to taste so awful that even neighborhood raccoons clawing through my garbage would take a pass.

From today onward, I will be some updated version of Dean. Today I'm Dean 2.0, later 3.0, etc. I will be like the *Rocky* franchise, with one key difference. I will be getting better with each new version, not worse. *Sorry Sly!*

4 ways to get your Beta on

1. Jump in now.

Inspiration is like milk. It comes with a best-if-used-by date and will expire if you wait until the cows come home. The longer you drag your feet, the more likely it becomes that your body transformation goals won't happen.

About two months after I started testing out ideas to lose weight, I discovered that I was actually putting on weight.

I immediately went online and started doing some research and came across something called the Paleolithic diet. I did a bit of research on it and was intrigued by the evolutionary aspect of the diet (more on this is Shift #1).

After about an hour of research, I was convinced it was worth a shot. I jumped on my bike, hit the neighborhood grocery store, and bought some paleo-type foods (i.e., meat). I started on the diet that night, immediately ending nineteen years of being vegetarian. I have never looked back.

It's one of the few times I just jumped in, as opposed to analyzing something to death and completely missing a great opportunity to **MAKE SHI**(F)**T HAPPEN**.

2. Design something to solve your own problem.

The best software programs out there happen because someone identifies a problem that doesn't have an elegant solution.

That's exactly the approach you must take with body transformation. Stop thinking someone else is going to solve your problem. Stop trying to use duct-tape-and-glue thinking, and instead design something that seamlessly works within your customized set of circumstances.

For instance, if you travel a lot, joining a gym is a not a great idea. You want something that could be done in your hotel room if need be. If you are a mother of two young children, you want a program that could be done when a thirty-minute block of time becomes available. A one-hour yoga DVD is not a practical solution.

Identify the challenges to your specific situation and then look to design something that accommodates them all.

MINDSET SHI(F)T: *37 Signals*

I'm a huge fan of 37 Signals. They are a leading software developer of products that help people and businesses effectively manage their projects.

However, they did not start out as a software developer. For the first five years of their existence, they were a website design company. One of the things they were struggling with was a way to effectively communicate with clients.

While there was project management software on the market, none of the available options adequately addressed the core issues they were struggling with, so they developed their own project management tool to help manage their design projects.

Soon clients started to ask if they could use it as well, and 37 Signals suddenly had a legitimate product on their hands that others could use.

In 2004 they released their project management tool and 37 Signals officially abandoned web design in favor of online web applications.

By choosing not to adopt a less adequate option, 37 Signals is now considered to be the one of best in the world at management software.

DO-IT-YOURSELF SHI(F)T:

If the solutions that currently exist do not address the problems you have, set about creating your own unique solution.

3. Embrace Simplicity.

"Simple rules lead to complex behavior. Complex rules, as with the tax law in most countries, lead to stupid behavior."

Andrew Hunt, *The Pragmatic Programmer*

Humans often like to take situations and make them horribly complex. I'm no exception, and in an effort to change my thinking, I decided to do the opposite and embrace simplicity.

I now require little to no equipment to work out. I eat the same meals day in and day out. I focus on a few key vital behaviors that have helped me generate results that I have never achieved in my previous forty-five years.

The more complex you make something, the less likely it can be sustained long-term. Adopt the principle of Occam's Razor—that the simplest explanation is the best one—to your lifestyle and pare things down.

4. Embrace constraints.

Most of us do the opposite. We complain about constraints and use them to justify our inactivity instead of embracing them as a set of parameters around which we can build our lives.

I hear constraints being used as excuses all the time. Here is a list of the most common refrains:

⇨ Eating healthy is too expensive.

⇨ I have no time.

⇨ I can't afford a gym membership.

⇨ I don't like to cook.

⇨ I get bored easily.

⇨ I travel a lot.

⇨ I have kids.

⇨ I don't have any home equipment for workouts.

⇨ I have (insert any ailment you can think of).

I have purposely created **shift** in my life by embracing some of the excuses people (me being one of them) use to avoid doing what they know they should be doing.

Everything I have created has been done…

⇒ On a limited budget (I was not working for a good stretch of my transformation).

⇒ With limited time (workouts *must* be thirty minutes or less).

⇒ With limited space (I work out in my living room, which is about the size of a Turkish prison cell).

⇒ With limited cooking skills.

⇒ Using limited equipment (I work with only six pieces of equipment).

⇒ Eating foods that are mostly not organic (a few are).

⇒ Eating meat that is not necessarily grass-fed.

MAKE SHI(F)T HAPPEN...

1 It's easy to come up with reasons why we can't do something. It's DAMN hard to acknowledge your constraints (some being very daunting) and still jump in. So enough of the excuses! It's time to get to work on Beta You now! Things won't be perfect (far from it, in fact), but remember that you can tweak and fix things for You 2.0.

COMMIT NOW TO JUMPING IN AND BEGIN TO CREATE BETA YOU!

---

2 Design something that specifically solves your problem. This book is a direct result of me solving my own problem.

Begin keeping your own notes and jotting down your own ideas and theories and test them out to see what works for you and what doesn't. This book came about by simply committing myself to writing out my own ideas and theories and then relentlessly testing them. Do the same.

WRITE YOUR MANUAL ON YOU!

---

3 Embrace simplicity. To learn more about simplicity, I would recommend you check out Leo Babauta, who is the author of the blog Zen Habits. Leo has a massive following (about 250,000 followers) and focuses on the art of simple living. There are many things you can borrow from Leo and apply on this journey.

www.zenhabits.net and www.leobabauta.com

REMEMBER, SIMPLICITY IS SUSTAINABLE. COMPLEXITY IS NOT.

LOG LIKE CAPTAIN KIRK ⇨

You have to love Captain Kirk. The guy was quite possibly the coolest television character ever created. But he was also one of the smarter ones, because he kept a log.

Every episode had him logging something that was crucial to the mandate of Star Fleet Command. Each log contained updates about missions and life forms the crew encountered (or in Kirk's case, life forms he made out with—seriously, the guy was an intergalactic horn dog).

The logging of information was crucial, as Kirk's data would form the foundation for future members of the Star Fleet in their quest to further explore the galaxy.

And while it's tempting to be put off by Kirk's fetish for alien chicks, there's a really valuable lesson to be learned from Captain K's ability to faithfully update the Star Fleet log.

But first let's discuss . . .

Why we get fat...

Here is my advantage that most "experts" don't have. I have lived five very distinct ways of eating. I expand on these more in Shift #1, but in sum I have eaten:

- A conventional government-approved diet (22 years)

- A no-red-meat diet (3 years)

- A vegetarian diet (14 years)

- A vegan diet (5 years)

- Ancestral or Paleolithic diet (most recent and by far the most successful for promoting optimal health for my body type)

The key word, of course, is *lived*. I have actually spent a considerable amount of time in each and have real results to back up my views.

Based on my own experience, I believe people are fat because . . .

They choose a way of eating that does not fit their particular body type.

Forget about citing studies and trying to impress people with scientific mumbo jumbo. People are simply eating in a way that does not allow their body to do what it is genetically bred to do (barring a medical condition to the contrary): *be lean*!

I realize people will take exception to the fact that I boiled this down to something so elementary. But the bottom line is that we have an obesity epidemic on our hands growing with each passing decade and yet people still spout the same useless rhetoric about weight-loss that they've been spouting for almost a century.

And you know what? It doesn't work!

Why we get fat 2.0...

If people are eating in a way that doesn't support their body type, then it is logical to assume that people get fat because they are consuming foods that are causing their bodies to store fat.

It's as simple as that.

If people want to achieve a state of leanness, then they need to devise a monitoring system to discover which foods are causing the damage.

Great bodies don't happen by accident...

It is only recently that I discovered that one of the vital behaviors of those who have a lean physique is that they carefully monitor what they put into their bodies.

There are a variety of ways to do this. Some log their foods using a software application, and others (a much smaller group) are so in tune with their body that they can innately monitor what they eat so that they are always in a state of optimal health.

One person that comes to mind is Mark Sisson of *Mark's Daily Apple* (www.marksdailyapple.com). Mark is fifty-eight (as of 2011) and has the body of a twenty-four-year-old beach volleyball player.

Let's not make the mistake of thinking this man is just genetically lucky. He hasn't always looked like that. He has done a tremendous amount of work so that he intuitively knows what he should be eating to put his body into an optimal state of health.

But for every Mark Sisson out there, there are thousands upon thousands who have awful bodies and subsequently awful health because they have no clue what they are eating or why they are eating it.

Sadly, these people have been *mindless eaters* their entire lives. I'm not casting stones here, because I was that mindless eater for forty-five years of my life.

MINDSET SHIFT: *Actor Jason Statham*

A number of years ago I read an article on the actor Jason Statham that mentioned he kept a journal with him at all times and wrote down everything that went into his mouth.

It should be noted that Statham is in awesome shape!

It dawned on me that a great physique does not happen by accident. One has to be very conscientious. I remember thinking that perhaps this was one of the key behaviors required to get the body we want.

THE RIGHT SHI(F)T: *Create a log*

The recording of my foods is the second-most-important behavior I adopted in this whole process (Shift #1 was my most important). By recording everything I eat, I make the invisible visible. That has been invaluable. So much so, in fact, that it's the first thing I tell clients to do when I start working with them. If you want to be conscientious about your eating, you first have to be aware of the food you put in your mouth, and keeping a log is the best way to be aware.

To log or not to log...

One of the harsh realities I had to come to grips with was the fact that I had no idea what foods I should and should not eat.

I had mistakenly assumed that eating "healthy" should lead to optimal health, but I had forty-five years of being me to prove that wasn't the case.

In fact, eating healthy was making me fatter.

If I was going to figure out what foods should be in my diet, I needed to start logging what I ate.

I had the same reservations as everyone else who doesn't currently log their foods: *This is going to be so much work*!

Here is how I convinced myself this was an experiment worth the investment:

On most really good days I can barely remember what I had for breakfast. If I am not logging my foods, how could I possibly know what I ate last week that might now be causing me to get fat today?

The answer—I wouldn't.

Understanding that it was unreasonable for me to think I could remember foods a week later without written documentation, I made the decision to attempt logging. I would relentlessly record the foods I ate and monitor how I was feeling so that I could begin to unlock the secrets to what foods actually worked for my body and which ones turned me into a disgusting blob of goo!

Finding a system that works...

When I finally opted into the idea of logging my foods, I used an Excel spreadsheet for the first few months. I quickly learned three things.

First, the mere act of recording what you eat makes you a more mindful eater.

Second, the act of writing down your foods is *not* enough. There is no data attached (such as a macronutrient breakdown), so the process is quite subjective. Subjective data is dangerous because most of us tend to draw simple and inaccurate conclusions, which end up doing us more harm than good. I needed data that I could actually comb through for clues and patterns.

Third, manually entering foods into Excel is time-consuming.

I decided to try a free online service. I used it for the next three months, and although it was extremely helpful, it was painfully slow and littered with distracting ads. *There is a reason free is free.*

I upgraded to a paid service instead, which gave me an automatic breakdown of both macronutrients (fats, carbohydrates, proteins, and calories) and micronutrients.

Here is a screenshot of a typical breakfast I have each morning.

Food Description	Brand	Servings		Meal
Avocados ~ California Raw		0.5	fruit	Breakfast
Coconut Oil Organic		1	tablespoon	Breakfast
Dandelion Greens Boiled ~ Drained ~ w/o Salt		0.5	cup, chopped	Breakfast
Eggs ~ Scrambled Whole Egg		3	eggs	Breakfast
Garlic ~ Organic Fresh		1	clove	Breakfast
Mushrooms Raw		0.5	cup, pieces or slices	Breakfast
Spinach Raw		0.75	cup	Breakfast
Tomatoes ~ Red Ripe ~ Raw ~ Year Round Average		0.5	cup, chopped or sliced	Breakfast

I like how quickly I can add what I have had along with the appropriate portion size. I do this for all the food I have in any particular day,
and it takes about five minutes. I mean, seriously, if I can't find five
minutes in my day to log the foods I am eating, then I have *much*
bigger issues than being fat.

From the diagram below you can see that I also get a macronutrient
breakdown of each meal. This data is crucial to my success. Actually,
there is only one number I really track that has been invaluable for
me (see Shift #2 to know what it is).

Food Summary

Meal	Calories	Fat	Carbs	Protein
Breakfast	271	27.1g	5.7g	5.7g
Snack #1	494	39.1g	12.5g	23.2g
Lunch	499	31.3g	23.9g	33.2g
Snack #2	420	32.0g	36.0g	8.0g
Dinner	154	2.8g	8.4g	23.8g
Snack #3	199	3.8g	7.0g	35.6g
Total Percentage of Calories [1]	**2037**	**136.1g** 58%	**93.5g** 18%	**129.5g** 24%

Going Sigmund Freud on yourself...

Simply tracking numbers is not enough if you are looking to create massive change. There are reasons why you do what you do, and if you aren't prepared to pull the bark off and see what is going on underneath the surface, then you will have little chance of succeeding in the long-term.

Here is an example of some notes I made for myself after having a tough day in the cravings department.

April 4, 2011: Fighting the junk food bug

Struggled most of the day with junk food cravings. What I am eating has not changed, but something interesting did happen this morning.

I was shooting video showing a typical breakfast I make myself. The only problem is I didn't eat that breakfast until 12PM. Normally I would eat it sometime between 8 and 9AM. I instead had walnuts during this time.

So my thinking is this: not having my normal controlled carb breakfast may have thrown my system off, causing the cravings I am battling.

I did not cave into these cravings, which is cool, but will work my butt off to make sure I don't deviate from my morning routine. But if I do, I will look to see if these cravings make an encore appearance. If so, then I now have one strategy to control them (the cravings).

MAKE SHI(F)T HAPPEN...

1 The key to weight-loss is to find the right combination of behaviors that will unlock the lean YOU desperately trying to get out. Tracking the foods you eat each and every day is one of those vital behaviors you must adopt.

There are many online software programs you can sign up for to start tracking what you are cramming into your belly. Pick something that works for you and your learning style.

RECORD AND MAKE THE INVISIBLE VISIBLE!

---

2 Pick one time each day where you will update your log. I choose to do mine first thing each morning when I log onto my computer. Treat it like you would a personal appointment.

I have mine scheduled in my iCal for 6:15 AM each morning. I get a message that pops up, reminding me the moment I log onto my computer. And I can't close the prompt until I have logged my foods and made my notes and observations.

HONOR YOUR FOOD LOG APPOINTMENT LIKE YOU WOULD A BUSINESS MEETING!

---

3 You don't need to log your foods for eternity (although it is a smart habit to maintain), but you should be prepared to do so for at least three to six months. I did it for an entire year before I felt I knew what I was doing. It is the smartest thing I have ever done.

IF YOU WANT TO CHANGE HOW YOU LOOK THEN TRACK WHAT YOU EAT!

RUN YOUR BODY LIKE YOU'D RUN A BUSINESS ⇨

Sometimes I find myself amid temptation. On a recent occasion it was a pack of scones bought by a friend and meant to share. Friends kept passing the plate around and offering me one. Every time they went by, I felt the scones staring at me, urging me to take a bite. The old me would have thought nothing of devouring one and licking the plate of any remaining crumbs. (Beware! That isn't a joke. I'm a plate-licker, so you may want to think twice about having me over for dinner.) Then again there was never a treat that the old me turned down, especially when it was free.

But these are different times and this is a different Dean (2.0!) so I let the scones pass me by.

What has changed?

Lots of things have changed. I know some are looking for one or two "quick" things they can use to mimic my success, but body transformation is a much more complicated process. How you eat and how you move are only two parts of a much larger puzzle you are attempting to solve to keep your body running smoothly.

Running your body like a great business…

I love *Fast Company* and *Inc.* magazines because I am fascinated with the idea of building a business around a lifestyle, and both of these publications do an excellent job profiling people who do just that. However, one of the things I have noticed is that a number of the people profiled and praised for their ability to run a great organization are in dire straits when it comes to their health. From a physical standpoint, a number of them are absolute train wrecks.

I found myself wondering why they didn't implement the same principles they use to lead their company to build a new and improved body.

Of course, as a fat guy myself at the time, I was not in a position to be offering weight-loss advice, but I understood that there were leadership principles required to run a successful business that also applied to running a successful body.

Striving for greatness…

Great companies don't stumble upon greatness. They deliberately set out to be great. They don't just set a goal, but rather carefully orchestrate the steps needed to reach it.

Google is a terrific example.

On their website they have a section where they share their business philosophy. It's pretty badass (sorry to go all gangsta' on you there) but, more importantly, it reinforces the notion that great things don't happen by accident.

Their philosophy is titled, "10 things we know to be true." Here are the ten guiding principles they use to govern how they do business:

1. Focus on the user and all else will follow.

2. It's best to do one thing really, really well.

3. Fast is better than slow.

4. Democracy on the web works.

5. You don't need to be at your desk to need an answer.

6. You can make money without doing evil.

7. There's always more information out there.

8. The need for information crosses all borders.

9. You can be serious without a suit.

10. Great just isn't good enough.

Google has become an epic company by having an epic philosophy.

This got me thinking, "Why should it be any different in the re-creating of my physique?"

Applying Google's business philosophy to my health.

I decided to build a personal philosophy to serve as a guide and make sure I stayed true to my values and my vision.

I would love to say that just-saying-no to the scones in the first paragraph was a typical example of "being disciplined" or using willpower, but that would be misinterpreting what happened— something many "experts" do.

It wasn't an act of discipline or willpower. **It was a matter of principle.**

I allow myself three treats per week on predetermined days (that week they happened to fall on Tuesday, Thursday, and Sunday). That particular day was a Saturday. It was not a treat day. I already knew what I was eating and that unexpected temptation was not on the roster.

Therefore, the decision to decline was simply an act of clarity.

Eating philosophy defined...

My current philosophy stands at twenty-five points and continues to evolve as I learn more about what works and doesn't work for me.

While twenty-five may seem excessive, my decision-making is improved significantly the more specific I am on the behaviors I expect from myself.

Here are some that have played more prominently in my success.

1. **Never be hungry.**
    A starvation diet is unsustainable and volatile, and it leads to binge eating and tremendous guilt.

2. **Eating must be enjoyable and functional.**
    There is a balance. Find it.

3. **Track everything I eat.**
   Tracking creates data. Data creates awareness. Awareness leads to smarter choices.

4. **Focus on simplicity.**
   Complexity is not sustainable in the long run. The more hoops you have to jump through, the more likely you are to get tripped up.

5. **Reward discipline.**
   Discipline without reward wanes. Treat myself three times a week on predetermined days and **honor** the process.

6. **Decide in advance.**
   Spontaneous decision-making usually defaults to actions that caused my problem in the first place.

7. **Eliminate the problem.**
   For me that meant no junk in the house, *ever.*

8. **Think sustainability.**
   Can I eat this way for the next five years? If not, it doesn't belong.

9. **Erase borders.**
   Create something that is *not* location specific. I should be able to easily adopt my eating whether on a camping trip, traveling, or locked in a Turkish prison (OK, maybe not that one).

10. **Ban permanently:**
    Supplements, chemically laden processed foods, grains, legumes, sugars, bad fats (I know this step seems like a really big one, but I'll further explain the benefits in Shift #1: Go paleo).

Movement philosophy defined...

My commitment to creating and following an eating philosophy was clearly working. I was making better choices more consistently than I had ever experienced before.

I decided to try the same approach with my workouts because working out without a clear action plan had been one of my major downfalls in the past. This time around I decided to take the business-prospectus-as-applied-to-my-body idea one step further.

Here is a sample of something I wrote in my journal on December 6, 2010, when I was rethinking my exercise program:

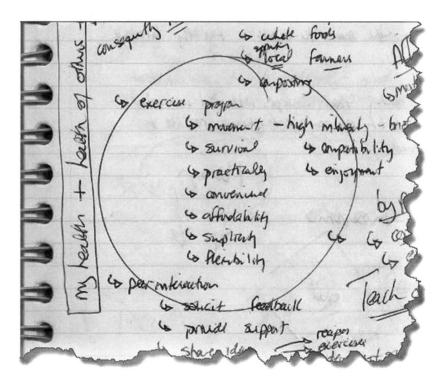

I apologize because clearly it seems I wrote that with my left foot. If you are not fluent in left foot, here is the translation of what I felt were the required elements in an epic exercise program:

- **Movement.**
  Incorporate a variety of movements at varying intensities, but *make it count*!

- **Survival.**
  Train so I could save a life or save my own if need be. Eliminate anything that doesn't help achieve that mandate (i.e., repetitive cardio).

- **Sustainability.**
  Time is a factor in a busy life. Keep programs at thirty minutes or less five times a week.

- **Convenience.**
  It can be done on my schedule or at a moment's notice.

- **Affordability.**
  No gym membership required.

- **Simplicity.**
  Equipment is not a precursor to a workout.

- **Flexibility.**
  I could do it anywhere within any space provided.

- **Compatibility.**
  It has to fit with my lifestyle at any particular moment in time.

- **Enjoyment.**
  Design it around stuff I like. Forced motivation is not sustainable long-term.

- **Creativity.**
  Design my own exercises; make my own equipment if need be.

- **Measurability.**
  Results must be measurable.

This was more than simply exercising to lose weight. My workouts were now a symbol of something much bigger and more epic, with a huge payoff in the end if done right.

BULLSHI(F)T: *Repetitive Cardio*

People (me included) have bought into this notion that we need to spend countless hours each week doing repetitive cardio like running or riding the stationary bike. There is little evidence to support that it leads to weight-loss.

Just take a look at runners. How many of us know people who have completed a marathon and yet look like they have not exercised a day in their life?

I'm not poking fun at these people, because most have trained long hours and damn hard in order to participate in these events. But people are under the illusion that these types of activities lead to weight-loss.

They do not. If they did, everyone who trained for a marathon would be in amazing shape.

THE RIGHT SHI(F)T: *Ditch the repetition*

Mindless plodding-type exercises do not lead to incredible transformation and should not be part of your program. Something that worked very well for me was adopting shorter workouts at high intensity. I accomplished this by reducing my rest time in between sets and increasing the number of reps and the amount of weight I used in subsequent workouts.

MAKE SHI(F)T HAPPEN...

1 If you are looking at making some BIG changes to your lifestyle, I strongly recommend creating an eating philosophy. Feel free to liberally use some of my principles but be sure to customize it to your body and circumstances.

For a copy of my eating philosophy, head over to
www.makeshifthappen.org/resources

A PHILOSOPHY CREATES CLEAR BOUNDARIES UPON WHICH TO OPERATE & EVALUATE!

2 The same holds true for developing an exercise program. Don't make the same mistake I made for twenty-five years. Doing stuff for the sake of doing stuff got me *nowhere*! If you want to create something epic, then take the time to think about what you want your program to do for you.

For a copy of my exercise philosophy head over to
www.makeshifthappen.org/resources

BOUNDARIES CREATE THE AWARENESS TO KNOW WHAT IS IN PLAY AND WHAT IS NOT!

3 Earlier I listed the ten things Google knows to be true, but on their site they go on to explain each in detail. It's a fascinating read. I have also included their ten things for a great user experience. Feel free to borrow from both as you create your philosophies.

Ten things Google knows to be true:
http://www.google.com/about/corporate/company/tenthings.html

Ten principles that contribute to a Google user experience:
www.google.com/about/corporate/company/ux.html

DETERMINE WHAT YOU KNOW TO BE TRUE!

SQUASH THE CHARACTER FLAW THEORY ⇨

One of the hardest things about trying to lose weight can be the sense of failure that comes when we have setbacks that keep us from reaching our goals. We take failure personally, attributing it to a character flaw— lack of discipline, lack of willpower, inability to see things through. The internal guilt trip can come up with endless personal shortcomings. A constant battle with weight creates psychological baggage. The baggage comes from a variety of sources, whether it's from the scrap heap of failed programs that we have tried and ultimately failed at or the mental beatings we give ourselves for lacking the discipline needed to lose weight.

Now, I would love to say that I have no emotional scars from my years of struggling with my weight, but that would be a big fat lie. The truth is, male or female, the emotional aspect of this journey plays a far more powerful role than any of us can imagine or care to admit.

If I was going to be honest with myself (and transformation *can't* happen until we are willing to be brutally honest), then I was going to have to confront the idea that years of mentally beating myself up for not reaching my health goals had left an imprint. Furthermore, I had to let go of the idea that my lack of results was caused by a flaw in my character.

When the universe intervenes . . .

Life is a pretty amazing thing. We work our butts off to impose our will on it. And yet sometimes, when we stop the struggle and just let life happen, serendipitous things occur.

In my particular case, life sent me a book that changed my view completely.

Someone had mentioned to me that our public library had recently installed software that would allow borrowers to download eBooks online.

I don't particularly enjoy going to the library. I have nothing against the library system, it's just that the last time I went someone stole the seat off my bike. It's kind of like someone stealing your toilet seat. You don't realize something is amiss until your butt hits water. It's much the same on a bike, only a bit more intrusive.

OK, where was I? Right, so I was browsing their eBook categories and saw that one of their featured books was *Why We Get Fat*. I was intrigued by the title of this book. Everyone addresses the outcome. Few have attempted to address the cause.

Unfortunately, the book was not available for download, so I checked out other books by the same guy.

It turns out Gary Taubes had another book, which was available, called *Good Calories, Bad Calories*. So I downloaded that and started reading it right away.

Two schools of thought . . .

First off, *Good Calories, Bad Calories* is *not Harry Potter* for fat people. It is not the kind of book you snuggle up with on a rainy day. The book has a very clinical feel to it. It's like reading a medical textbook while in a hospital gown with a thermometer sticking out of your bum.

However, there were a few ideas Taubes mentions that just blew me away:

The first was the realization that I needed to learn to make the distinction between good science vs. bad science. There is *a lot* of bad science out there, and many of us (myself included) blindly accept something simply because there was a study done or some so-called expert said it was so.

> ## BULLSHI(F)T:
> ### *When good people believe stupid things*
>
> When I was twelve, a friend accidentally burned down his garage and set his leg on fire at the same time. My brother and I eventually got his leg to stop burning, but he now had a serious burn on his leg. We watched in horror/amusement as one of our neighbors jumped into action and smothered the leg in toothpaste to help "heal" the burn.
>
> Now I was no baby Einstein, but even at age twelve I knew that toothpaste would not heal a burn. That was about the silliest thing you could put on it, next to maybe barbeque sauce, which at least would have been thematically appropriate based on the situation. But the neighbor had heard somewhere that toothpaste was a good thing to put on a burn and took that to be fact without ever questioning the source.
>
> ## THE RIGHT SHI(F)T: *Question the source*
>
> We need to be far more critical of the information we decide to accept as fact. Just because someone says so or a study is cited does not make it any less wrong or stupid. Before you accept something as fact, question the source: What are the expert's credentials? What were the parameters of the study cited? Was the data interpreted correctly?

The second big idea I learned from Taubes's book was that there were two schools of thought on obesity. There were those who believed that it was caused by underactivity and overeating. And there was a much smaller group who thought there had to be another explanation.

Based on my own experience, I no longer subscribed to the former. I was a perfect example of someone who watched what he ate and worked out pretty intensely four or five days a week. In practice this theory held no validity for me. If it was as simple as that, then I should have been Lean Dean. There had to be another reason why it looked like I had eaten Lean Dean.

A "What if" for the ages . . .

About halfway through the book, I stumbled upon a rather obscure idea:

WHAT IF WEIGHT GAIN IS A SYMPTOM OF SOMETHING THAT HAS GONE WRONG WITH OUR BODY ON A CELLULAR LEVEL?

It was a holy shi(f)t moment. I had *never* heard weight gain presented in this context.

My poor little brain didn't know what do. I could hear it screaming, "Is this even plausible?"

I started thinking about people I had known who had undergone rapid weight gain over a few short years. You know the people I am talking about. We don't see them for a while and then when we do our inner heckler says, "Holy sweet baby Jesus, what the hell happened to you?"

The standard argument is that these people have embraced the dark side and are now consuming more calories than they are burning.

I suspect that is possible, but surely that can't be true in all cases. Was it not possible that perhaps something happened on a cellular level that caused their cells to no longer be as efficient as they once were?

It seemed logical to me that this was in fact plausible. What if their cells, which had been extremely efficient at processing all the crap they were consuming over the years, suddenly hit a speed bump and were no longer functioning at 100 percent efficiency?

A paradigm shift emerges . . .

For the first time in my forty-five years, I had the elementary beginnings of a hypothesis I wanted to test. For starters, I needed a way to visualize what might be occurring on a cellular level and what I could do to help my cells out.

That's when I drew inspiration from an unlikely source: the Dyson vacuum cleaner (more on that in Shift #13).

MAKE SHI(F)T HAPPEN...

1 Reframe the way you see weight gain by embracing the possibility that weight gain is a symptom and not a character flaw, thus opening up the possibility to begin the process of rebuilding something that has suffered serious structural damage: your self-esteem.

Seriously, think about what it means if weight gain is not caused by a flaw in your personality. How does that change just about everything you have thought about yourself? The implications of this are immense.

WHEN YOU REFRAME THE PROBLEM YOU ALLOW FOR UNDISCOVERED SOLUTIONS!

---

2 Let's assume that your weight gain is a symptom of something that has gone wrong on a cellular level and not a character flaw. How can embracing this notion dramatically change your life?

Let me help you frame this by sharing my own breakthroughs. I realized that:

⇨ **I did not lack discipline.**

What really happened was I had simply opted out of stuff that wasn't working, which is what every normal person does when something isn't working, whether it is a job, a relationship, or a way of eating.

⇨ **My weight gain was an SOS message from my cells.**

Gaining weight was my cells' way of saying, "Dude, help us! We are trying to keep you lean, but we are completely outnumbered." So the question shifted from *What is wrong with me?* to *How can I help my cells do their job more effectively?*

⇨ **I had to stop beating myself up thinking I was a failure.**

I was not a failure. My cells were failing. That's a big freaking distinction!

WHAT ASSUMPTIONS HAVE YOU MADE ABOUT YOU THAT NOW MIGHT BE WRONG?

3 Many of your problems may be the result of false assumptions you have made about yourself. On the worksheet provided, actually sit down and identify some of these assumptions you have made and how they have shaped the old you. Now how can you reframe them to help shape the new lean you?

Challenging your assumptions worksheet:
www.makeshifthappen.org/resources

CHANGE HOW YOU LOOK BY CHANGING HOW YOU THINK ABOUT YOU!

CREATE
A VACUUM ⇨

What if, as I learned in the last chapter, **obesity was a symptom or side effect and not a character flaw?**

Now as much as I knew this "what if" question was going to have a monumental impact on reshaping how I perceived my weight problem, I was still unsure how to actually use this information.

As previously mentioned, I am very much a visual learner. While I understand most things on an intellectual level, if I don't have a clear picture of what an idea might look like, I am unable to create an action plan based on said idea.

In this case I had a theory but knew I had to find a way to visualize it in order to help me fully grasp the enormity of my newfound discovery. I understood that this discovery was going to allow me to take action; I just needed to figure out what that action was.

Answers come in the most unlikely of places . . .

Humans are a complex species. We are always seeking solutions to the questions we have, *except* we regularly fail to see them (the solutions) because we expect life to smack us upside the head with those answers.

For me, the solution came while reading the autobiography of James Dyson.

That's right, James Dyson, the inventor of the Dyson vacuum cleaner. You might even own one yourself.

His vacuums are spectacular. In fact, I would go so far as to say he is the Steve Jobs of the vacuum cleaner world. He has crafted a design that is stunning in its appearance (I would boldly refer to it as art), exceptional in its craftsmanship, and legendary in its technology (the first to apply cyclone technology to a vacuum cleaner).

If you are looking to be inspired by someone who truly personifies perseverance, then I highly recommend you get yourself a copy of *Against All Odds*. His story is truly incredible.

MINDSHIFT:
Why character traits are not possessions

I mentioned in previous shifts that many people don't understand their own success. Nowhere is this more evident than in how they talk about the character traits needed to succeed.

Most make the mistake of simply listing off a few traits they consider to be keys to success as things to have or have not. The problem is they make them sound like items you pick off the shelves at the nearest Character Trait Store and drop in your shopping cart.

Confidence—check

Perseverance—check

Hard work—check

But you don't "**have**" these character traits. You build each one from the ground up, a platform at a time with each small success you experience.

Case in point: James Dyson. He spent five years and developed 5,127 prototypes before the first bag-free vacuum cleaner was introduced to the world.

Some would say he succeeded because he *had* perseverance. I would disagree strongly with that. He didn't possess perseverance; he *nurtured* his ability to persevere one prototype at a time.

It helps to envision character traits evolving as a series of platforms that stack upon each other like Legos. In Dyson's case, the first prototype gave him the confidence to build a platform to reach for the second. The second gave a platform to reach for the third, and so on. Each subsequent platform was built on the previous platforms. The same can be said of traits like confidence, willpower, and the like.

Yes there will be setbacks along the way. There will be times when you fall off a platform you have built. It happens. That's how character traits evolve. But only when you understand the process do you understand how to pick yourself up, brush yourself off, and begin to rebuild your platform.

THE RIGHT SHI(F)T: *Build a platform*

Body transformation requires the same prototypical approach. You don't get the body you want on the first try. But each successive prototype helps you expand on your platforms. And like James Dyson, at some point a critical mass of platforms are present and that's when success occurs.

When NOT SUCKING sucks...

I was actually reading Dyson's autobiography for the second time. I had read it about five or six years ago, and for some unknown reason the book seemed to be calling out to me again, so I plucked it off my bookshelf and began re-reading his story.

Of course, like all books I read, I had forgotten pretty much everything I read the first time around. Unfortunately, my memory has a hard time remembering its job . . . FYI memory . . . it is to *remember* stuff.

Anyhow, I love stories, and Dyson was recounting how he came to start tinkering with the idea of creating a better, more efficient vacuum cleaner.

His vacuum cleaner at the time worked using bag technology, and for any of us who still use this outdated piece of crap technology (I am one of them sadly), then you know that over time the vacuum becomes less and less efficient.

Dyson was having the same issue. His vacuum cleaner kept losing suction after each subsequent use, so one day he finally had enough and ripped the bag off to understand the internal dynamics of the thing.

The anatomy of vacuum bag technology...

The vacuum cleaner is the quintessential household item, and yet the nuts-and-bolts of how it works were alien to me. Allow me to give you the Cliff Notes version on how a vacuum cleaner works.

When you turn the vacuum on, air is sucked through the nozzle into the inner sanctum of the vacuum cleaner. As you pass it over the floor it sucks up dirt, pennies, receipts, small family heirlooms, and other important crap we didn't know we had dropped, but still need, and sadly will never see again.

Here's the part I had never taken the time to understand: It turns out that a vacuum cleaner bag is much like our skin in that it is equipped with pores. In the case of the vacuum, air and dirt are sucked in and the air then escapes through these tiny pores, while the dirt (larger than the pores) is trapped inside the bag.

This sounds brilliant, but here is the problem. Over time, the pores of the bag get clogged by the dirt being sucked in, thus decreasing the exit efficiency for the air molecules. Put another way, if Elvis was the air, he would have a hard time leaving the building.

This creates a bottleneck, as the air molecules currently in the system take longer to exit. It functions exactly the same way rush hour traffic does. When the volume of traffic exceeds the holding capacity of the highway system, everything slows down to a crawl.

That's exactly what happens in the vacuum. As more and more of the pores get plugged with dirt, the number of viable exits dwindles, and the system is no longer able to manage the sheer volume of air that is still being pumped into the system.

More and more suction is lost over the life of a bag until it is no longer sucking up anything. And for vacuum cleaners, *not* sucking sucks.

In reality, the only way to ensure high-quality suction with a vacuum cleaner that uses bag technology is to change the bag long before it's full, which is terribly inefficient and not very environmental.

This was the problem that Dyson set out to solve.

Extending an idea...

I was captivated by this story for two reasons. One, the more I understand how something works, the more ways I can find to extend the ideas to other areas of my life. Second, I thought I could use it at parties to impress women.

While I vastly overestimated how mesmerized the ladies would be by my vacuum cleaner prowess, it did have a profound impact on my journey to a better body, because a few days later it hit me.

What if my cells are like a vacuum cleaner bag? What if, over time, they had become clogged and were simply unable to do their job as efficiently as they once did?

This was precisely the visual connection I needed to help me understand the problem at hand.

If my weight gain was a side effect of something gone wrong on a cellular level, was it possible that my cells were simply too clogged up to be able to do their job efficiently? This job, of course, was the ability to eliminate fat from my body.

If this was so, then my job was to figure out how to allow them to do their job more efficiently. My mission (which I chose to accept) was to figure out what foods were causing my cells to crap out on me when I needed them most.

While this might not seem like a monumental discovery, this was HUGE for me. For the first time ever, I had a working theory about why I was the way I was, with a clear and simple analogy to explain it.

This was my James Dyson "rip the bag off the vacuum cleaner" moment. I now had a mission that thankfully had nothing to do with the conventional (and short-sighted) wisdom about weight-loss.

MAKE SHI(F)T HAPPEN...

1 There will be lots of "smart" people in lousy shape that will be eager to convince you this idea is not plausible. I urge you to think for yourself and decide whether this is an idea worth adopting. Consider the possibility that there are foods you eat that are overwhelming your cells and preventing them from doing their job . . . *to keep you lean.*

EXPOSE YOURSELF TO THE IDEAS OF OTHERS, BUT THINK FOR YOURSELF.

---

2 What foods do you think are preventing you from being lean? Go beyond the obvious ones. I mention in an upcoming shift that I learned beans made me fat. Adding that to my growing list of foods I could not eat helped my cells do their intended job . . . to get me lean.

Start a list and begin testing to see what is making you fat.

WHAT FOODS ARE PREVENTING YOU FROM BEING LEAN?

---

3 Weight-loss is a horrible industry. There is a lot of bad information out there that doesn't make it any less bad because many people believe it. It took one man five years to believe there was a better way to build a vacuum cleaner.

WHAT ARE YOU WILLING TO BELIEVE TO BUILD YOURSELF A BETTER BODY?

DECLARE WAR ON RESISTANCE

What I am about to address goes by many names. Bible enthusiasts refer to it as temptation brought on by the landlord of Hell. Freud referred to it as the ego. In *Linchpin*, Seth Godin calls it our lizard brain. And our fictional friend Obi-Wan Kenobi referred to it as "The Dark Side."

But author Steven Pressfield captures it best when, in his book *The War of Art,* he referred to it as "resistance."

What is resistance?

Resistance is that voice inside your head (our inner heckler) that just won't shut up. It is that voice that attempts to sabotage every worthwhile adventure you launch.

Pressfield says,

> Resistance is the most toxic force on the planet. It is the root of more unhappiness than poverty, disease and erectile dysfunction. To yield to resistance deforms our spirit. It stunts us and makes us less than we are and were born to be.

My battle with resistance . . .

To be honest, the notion of resistance was not even on my radar when I first started this new journey. In fact, it never has been. I was always preoccupied with fat loss and getting a damn six-pack. What foods was I going to eat? How would I track them? What exercises was I going to perform? How often would I work out and for what duration?

These were my primary concerns as I began to embark on yet another fat-loss effort. But as I ventured forth, I was struck with the notion that my real battle seemed *not* to be with my body fat, but rather with this thing I had yet to officially identify; this mammoth, ugly soul-sucking creature that lurked within the shadows of my psyche—my own version of resistance.

It seems so elementary now (Watson, are you there?), but resistance has always been my issue.

As I began to comb through the scrap heap of past failures, I could see resistance would:

- Keep me from doing the research I needed to do to find a specific solution geared to my body-type.

- Encourage me to skip a workout, saying I had earned it.

- Push me to hit the corner store and support the Ben and Jerry's fat foundation when I was feeling lousy about something.

- Tell me that what I was doing wasn't working and that it was time to abandon this foolishness.

- Hit the snooze button for the umpteenth time.

- Shout back from the mirror, "Dude, you don't have the genetics to be thin. Stop this nonsense!"

Resistance is smart. Damn smart!

The thing about resistance is that it is really freaking clever. Well, at least mine is. It does its best to keep the status quo, but it also knows when it needs to throw me a bone so it won't lose me.

This is what it would do.

It would let me get all excited about a new program. It would let novelty have the stage and run the show for a few weeks, a month, sometimes even three or four months.

Then, with its critics-eye-view, it would start to submit its reviews on my latest program.

- "A colossal waste of time," came one.
- "A great stocking stuffer for those running low on crap that doesn't work" another review would say.
- "It's just like getting something for nothing except in this case you are getting nothing for something," came another.

OK, that is not exactly how my resistance talks to me, but you get the gist of the messages it bombards me with every single day.

This is what had controlled me for years.

If I was going to change the very fabric of my future, I needed to recognize that resistance was my opponent and we were locked in something bigger than a battle. This was a full-on war where death to the enemy was the only solution.

Location, location, location . . .

To fight resistance, it helps to know where it lives. There is nothing more humiliating than suiting up for battle, renting a horse, and arriving at the wrong battle scene.

And Google Maps can't help you with this search. Well, it can, but it takes you to France, and, well, that is the wrong Resistance. Really, try it yourself and see.

Resistance lives in the gap between the body you have and the body you want. (Disclaimer: While I did draw these fictional characters myself, any resemblance to anyone you might know is purely coincidental.)

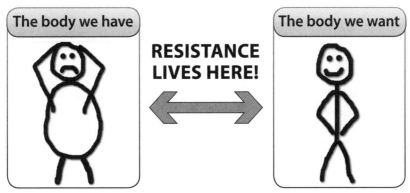

And that gap is like a moat around an ancient castle, infested with crocs and dragons. (Sorry, this is my story and this moat has dragons. Deal with it!)

Navigating the gap is treacherous and littered with the corpses of past YOUs who bravely, but naively, tried to pass, thinking nothing more than determination would keep you above water.

I have learned the hard way on this one. Determination makes for a lousy flotation device.

Reality check . . .

Strong in all of us resistance is (that's my inner Yoda talking), and if we are not equipped to do battle, it will beat us to an emotional pulp.

But it is really important to note that from time to time resistance is going to win a battle here-and-there, even when our intentions are to the contrary.

There will be days when resistance kicks the shi(f)t out of you and you relapse into old, familiar, and horribly ineffective habits that hinder your progress.

And when this happens, here is the most important lesson to remember.

Never rationalize your behavior. Recognize that you had a setback and move on.

BULLSHI(F)T: *Experts never struggle*

I am not a big fan of experts, simply because most are so desperate to come off as an expert that they create this illusion that they have everything figured out; that they don't ever struggle with anything.

This is ridiculous, of course. They still have struggles. The difference now is they have better strategies in place to silence their resistance when it tries to make its voice heard. And if they do experience a rare moment of weakness, they quickly go into recovery mode to immediately get themselves back on track.

I am no exception. Sometimes I eat things I shouldn't. Just to be clear here, I am referring to unhealthy foods as opposed to things like dental floss, shoelaces, or tin foil. Obviously, I wish this wouldn't happen, but it does, and it will continue to happen periodically.

The difference now is that it happens very infrequently, and when it does, I know how to minimize the damage by going into recovery mode. And the great news is, those are all learned skills (which I didn't possess when I was fat) that can be adopted by anyone.

THE RIGHT SHI(F)T: *Everyone struggles; learn to embrace it and cope with it*

Lose the notion that you will never struggle. You will. That's normal. Instead, embrace the idea that all you lack are the coping skills and strategies needed to help you deal with resistance, control the damage, and get back on course quickly.

The reasons rationalization is deadly...

Rationalization is a tool resistance uses to help you justify your actions. The moment you listen to resistance's rationale is the moment you put yourself on the fast track to complete and utter failure.

Why?

First, it eliminates personal accountability. It completely lets you off the hook for behavior that isn't congruent with what you want.

Second, it disguises the fact that you failed.

And third, rationalization displaces problem solving. The two cannot coincide within the same space. One is heads to the other's tails. When you seek to make excuses, you are rationalizing. By default, problem solving is disengaged.

The silver lining is that the reverse is also true. When you seek the truth, the brutal honest truth, you engage in problem solving, solution finding, and universal intelligence.

BULLSHI(F)T: *Two weeks' notice*

I had someone on Twitter comment that they liked my blog. When I checked out his profile, I could see from his headshot that he was easily fifty to eighty pounds overweight. I was curious to know if he was actually on the paleo diet or not so I tweeted back and asked.

He said he was "probably" going to start in two weeks.

Two weeks! I remember thinking, "WTF! Is he giving the food pyramid governing body two weeks' notice? Does he need to give them time to find a replacement?"

I have since learned that anyone who is going to start on "this date" is actually looking to find reasons why they can't do something. I decided to send this follow-up tweet to see how this guy was going to rationalize his decision.

 beingprimal Dean Dwyer
@█████ Just curious why you are waiting 2 weeks to start? What's keeping you from giving it go right now?
15 Aug

His response: That was when he and his wife would be going grocery shopping.

Unless you live in an underground bunker that is sealed for two-week stretches, that's just a lame-o reason to postpone beginning the process of reclaiming your body and your life.

THE RIGHT SHI(F)T IS RIGHT NOW

Unless you are in a coma, change should start *now*! When you look to postpone something, you're letting resistance do the talking, and it's hoping to buy time to find reasons why you shouldn't do this.

MAKE SHI(F)T HAPPEN...

1 Rationalization is easily recognized in the things we say to others or in the chatter that goes on inside our noggins. Here are five common things people say that you should be especially wary of. While there might be some truth that exists when any of those statements are uttered, it is your resistance talking and looking for ways to cover up your failings.

1. Well, it could have been worse.

This hides the fact that failure occurred. A small failure or a big failure is irrelevant. It's still failure. Don't water it down by indicating it could have been worse because, you know what, it could have been better.

Shift: Take ownership for your failure and analyze what went wrong. Those who succeed at getting and maintaining a state of leanness do so because they quickly diagnose their failures by identifying **specific** behaviors that didn't happen.

These include things such as "I didn't decide in advance," "I didn't plan in advance," or "I was not emotionally prepared to deal with that particular situation."

2. I worked out today so I can eat this.

This is one of the stupidest things I used to say. Most people don't realize how few calories most of our activities actually burn. As a result, the crap we give ourselves permission to eat cancels out our workout and leaves us at a caloric surplus. Translation: You just made yourself fatter.

Shift: Never trade off a workout for a bad-eating decision.

3. What the hell, you only live once.

This very misleading statement is missing one adjective. It omits how well you live that one life. I have seen some live a **horrible** life once. I have seen others thrive at life once. There are two sides to every coin. Which would you rather be on?

Shift: Flip the coin: use the same line of thinking to turn down things that negatively impact the quality of your life.

4. I'm better than I used to be.

This isn't about what you used to be, it's about who you are striving to be. You are either being who you want to be or you are not. Being a slightly better version of the old you is like saying, "I suck much less than I used to."

Shift: Imagine how your life would be different if you started saying, "No thank you. I want to be more than I am now."

5. I will begin in "X" days, weeks, or months.

This is exactly how people who fail to take action talk. It gives the illusion change is on the horizon without actually doing anything. What is really happening is that resistance is trying to buy some time to find reasons why you shouldn't be doing "this."

Shift: Start *now*! Resistance can't exist in the presence of immediate action.

WATCH YOUR LANGUAGE!

2 Start with something small. In fact, when you are trying to create massive change, taking smaller bites to start is a great way to build confidence. Here are three ideas to get you started:

⇨ eating a great breakfast for the next thirty days

⇨ signing up for an online food-tracking service and simply starting to record what you eat every single day

⇨ deciding to remove sugar from your coffee

START NOW! THINK SMALL! BUT DO SOMETHING!

---

3 The more you know about resistance, the greater your success in dealing with it. Below are two books that deal with resistance and are well worth the read:

The War of Art by Steven Pressfield (www.stevenpressfield.com)

Linchpin by Seth Godin (www.sethgodin.com)

CONSTANTLY SEEK TO BUILD YOUR LIBRARY OF SUCCESS!

Shift #11
LOSE YOUR MINDLESSNESS

Would you believe me if I were to tell you that we make roughly 200+ eating-related decisions each and every day? That's a crap-load of decisions, and that's only about food. I'm not counting all the other decisions we make daily in all the other areas of our life.

Now I need to give props where props are due. I actually hijacked that piece of trivia from Dr. Brian Wansink, who is the author of *Mindless Eating: Why We Eat More Than We Think.*

Not tested on animals...

Wansink and his team study how elements of our physical environment impact our eating behavior. Here is the kicker. He doesn't do research on rats or monkeys or Tasmanian devils. He studies a species that is highly volatile and extremely difficult to predict—*humans*!

Yes, that's right. He actually conducts his studies using real live people while testing various influences to see how they might respond.

MINDSHIFT: ½ *lb of M&M's vs. 1 lb of M&M's*

Wansink was curious to know whether portion size impacts how much we eat. So here is what he did.

He chose forty parents who were going to attend a PTA meeting. During this meeting they would be watching a video. The content of the video was irrelevant to the study. He just wanted something that would draw their attention away from the food they were eating.

They were then divided into two groups of twenty. The first group got a half-pound bag of M&M's. The other got a one-pound bag.

After the video was over, the bags were collected and the number of M&M's eaten were counted.

On average, the people with the half-pound bag ate 71 M&M's. The people with the one-pound bag ate 137 M&M's. If you forgot to bring your abacus with you, let me help you out.

The people who had twice as many M&M's ate nearly twice as much.

> **THE RIGHT SHI**(F)**T:** *Controlling availability leads to portion control*
>
> Don't eat M&Ms, for starters, unless being fat is your goal. Further to that, portion size will influence how much you eat. The more you have, the more you will mindlessly eat.

200...

I typically ignore most studies that cross my path for a host of reasons, but the one that Wansink conducted to determine the number of decisions we make each day about food really captured my attention.

Two hundred—that's a lot of decisions. That's one decision every four minutes and forty-eight seconds if you factor out sleeping hours (although I probably make food decisions in my sleep, I don't act on them). That's a ton of decisions to make about what to cram into your mouth.

Honestly, I thought of this study often when I began my journey. And I even took the liberty to craft my own theory as to why we make so many decisions in this area.

People have no clue what they are going to eat each day.

For a large percentage of the population, each meal is a complete mystery, waiting to be stumbled upon, driven to, or plucked from the nearest vending machine; even when to eat is a mystery.

Of course, this is a recipe for disaster and precisely why most people are fat.

AWARENESS SHIFT: *Did you know?*

Wansink conducted other studies. In one study it showed that, on average, when people ate with:

- 1 other person: **they ate 35% more**
- 4 other people: **they ate 75% more**
- 7 or more people: **they ate 96% more**

THE RIGHT SHI(F)**T:** *Make it your business to know or you'll succumb to outside influence*

Peer pressure is not something we only experience as kids. We are still influenced by it now. But what is worse this time around is we are not aware of it. Make it your business to understand where external pressure comes from and the pressure within will be the only influence.

The weight (pun intended) of decision making...

What people fail to recognize is that decisions are often heavy, grueling, and time-consuming. The sheer volume of decisions that we are constantly and unknowingly making can and often does suck the life out of us over the course of any given day. Do you really want to be deciding what and when to eat every five minutes of your waking hours?

Add stress or simply the many other things we have to think about everyday and we enhance the probability that when it comes to making our food choices, we will simply flip a switch and launch into default mode.

What is default mode? This is where we mindlessly choose something to eat that is quick, easy, accessible, and usually completely unhealthy for us.

Having been a victim of this pattern for most of my life, I needed to squash the ambiguity that existed when it came to making choices about what I ate. It was making me fat.

So I came up with a rather bold goal.

Zero decisions?

Resistance loves indecision. It craves it. It sits lurking in a corner waiting for a moment when I am indecisive and, when that moment arrives, it leaps in with reckless abandon to fill in the gap left by my befuddled mind.

I figured that if I want to change how I looked, I needed to drastically reduce the number of decisions surrounding the what, when, and where to eat.

Then it hit me. What if I didn't have to make any decisions about what I ate?

I know that seems both naive and ambitious, but I felt that I had an easy and manageable three-part solution to drastically cut down on, if not completely eliminate, food-related decisions.

First, I would create an eating philosophy. This would include a set of criteria that would frame how I was going to eat and why (as discussed in Shift #15).

Second, I would map out exactly what a great eating day would look like.

I decided in advance that I would eat six meals each day and that each meal would be constructed around a theme.

Having a theme upon which to structure meals would automatically make my eating a very *mindful* process while drastically reducing the number of decisions I was required to make.

Meal #1 . . .

Good healthy fat

Good clean carbs

Lean protein source

Breakfast truly is the most important meal of my day. The foundation for this meal is almost always eggs. The good, clean carbs come from a variety of fresh, seasonal, and local vegetables. I also include one or two healthy fats, which could be avocado on the side along with a healthy coconut or olive oil.

Snack #1 . . .

Raw nut mix

This typically tends to be raw almonds. I like them because they are a wonderful blend of healthy fat, protein, and carbs, and there's no prep time.

Meal #2 . . .

Good healthy fat

Good clean carbs

Lean protein source

Typically, I have a MONSTER salad here. The lean protein source could be canned tuna or salmon, and on occasion grilled chicken, sausage, turkey, or other meat (lots of great options that can be added for variety). I add a ton of fresh, *raw* veggies and top it off with a homemade dressing.

Snack #2 . . .

Veggies with nut butter

Raw nut mix

Celery and carrot sticks with almond butter are an absolute favorite of mine.

Meal #3 . . .

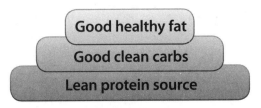

This varies. Sometimes I have eggs again. Beef stir-fries are very common here as well, with a boatload of good, clean carb sources, raw and cooked. The philosophy stays the same, but the options are endless.

Snack #3 . . .

Fruit with cinnamon

I don't have this every night, but a nice bowl of blueberries (frozen are surprisingly tasty) or strawberries with cinnamon is a very tasty treat. I like the fact that my last meal is low in fat, as it seems to flush my system so that when I awake in the morning I feel clean and lean.

Plan the work and work the plan...

Third, I created a weekly plan where I would know exactly what I would eat each day at each meal.

What this enables me to do is plan my entire week meal-by-meal so that in the moment I have no thinking to do whatsoever. So Monday night meal #3 will be Beef Stir-Fry. Meal #2 for Thursday afternoon will be a Monster Tuna Salad.

You get the picture here. By having a clear-cut philosophy on how I am going to approach meals and deciding in advance what I am going to eat, I eliminate almost all the decisions I am required to make throughout the day.

People would be amazed how easy it is to be disciplined when we already know what we are going to eat.

MAKE SHI(F)T HAPPEN...

1 Get Wansink's book *Mindless Eating: Why We Eat More Than We Think*. But don't just read it. Study it. Underline important passages. Scribble notes in the margins. Write out key ideas you discover. Make this your bible to becoming a more mindful eater.

LEARN TO BE MINDFUL OF WHAT YOU EAT!

2 Decide how many meals you will have each day and fill in how a typical eating day will look for you. Remember the more you fly by the seat of your pants, the larger that seat becomes. (Translation: your ass grows in proportion to the amount of time you wing it with your eating!)

GREAT HEALTH IS LIKE A BIG ASS. NEITHER HAPPENS BY ACCIDENT!

3 Go back and complete your damn eating philosophy from Shift #15. Don't make me have to tell you again. It is easy to put this off. Hell, I put mine off for twenty-five years but I'm telling you, it makes a tremendous difference, especially in the area of becoming mindful of what you eat.

AN EATING PHILOSOPHY IS CRITICAL TO MINDFULNESS AND GETTING LEAN!

BE BRUTALLY HONEST ⇨

This much I have learned. I don't care what part of your life you are trying to change, if you are not prepared to be completely honest about your current situation and why you are where you are, you can forget about getting to where you want to be.

That is so important to the process that it is worth repeating.

It is **IMPOSSIBLE** to achieve seismic transformational change until you are prepared to be brutally honest about your circumstances as they currently exist.

MINDSET SHIFT: *Reframe the issue*

The biggest mistake people make is framing their struggles with weight as a weight-loss issue. It's not! It is an issue of personal leadership.

As such, I encourage you to focus less of your efforts on weight-loss resources and lean on resources that focus on the core principles of leadership and change.

THE RIGHT SHI(F)T: *Take inspiration from sources that inspired you*

The principles required to take a business from good to great are exactly the same required to take a body from ho-hum to awesome!

Try this: go through your bookshelf and pull out one book you have read before that had a great impact on you (preferably nonfiction). Read it again and look for principles to apply to your own journey. I guarantee you will find some, regardless of the topic of the book.

Good to great...

I would love to say this shift is an original, but the truth is I got this idea from Jim Collins and his book *Good to Great*.

I am always looking for great ideas from unlikely sources. Not unlikely because they are obscure (Jim Collins is a huge bestselling author), but unlikely because they might focus on an issue that doesn't feel relevant to someone tackling a completely different issue.

For instance, in *Good to Great,* Jim Collins writes about how companies can make the leap from good to great. Someone battling weight-loss might not look to Jim Collins because his area of expertise is business, not weight-loss. I'd argue that Jim Collins's advice could be invaluable to those who want to take their bodies from good to great, or even from not-so-good to great. He's not only a business expert, he's a change expert, and with a little applied thinking you can transfer his advice to anything you think needs changing.

All of the books and personalities I've mentioned here may not be considered weight-loss sources in the traditional sense, but I believe they all have something to bring to the table. Part of my goal with this book is to help you see how you can draw inspiration and ideas for your own weight-loss goals from many places outside the weight-loss industry. Draw inspiration from areas you naturally enjoy. I personally love stories of transformation, so whenever I hear about a book that focuses on amazing change I always make a note of checking it out.

In this case, a guy I follow online, Chris Guillebeau (whom I mentioned back in Shift #19), happened to rave about Collins and his book. Because I have much respect for Chris and what he does (the guy is pretty freaking trustworthy), I picked up a copy of the book.

It did not disappoint.

The Stockdale Paradox.

There is a reason *Good to Great* has sold over four million copies. It's pure gold. Better yet, there are tons of ideas for crafty people to apply to their own situations.

One of those ideas was this: *brutal honesty.*

Collins and his team found that one of the key behaviors found in the eleven companies they researched for their ability to transition from good to great was their willingness to confront the most brutal facts of their situation.

He referred to it as the Stockdale Paradox, aptly named after Admiral Jim Stockdale.

Stockdale's tale . . .

Stockdale's story was unbelievable. He was a Vietnam POW from 1968 to 1975. He'd spent eight years of his life as a prisoner of war. To help put this in perspective, Stockdale passed away at the age of 81, so he was a POW for roughly 10 percent of his life.

Collins met up with him many years after his experience to ask him how he was able to survive repeated tortures and the notion that he had no idea if he would ever get out alive.

He attributed his ability to survive to two things. One was unwavering faith that he would one day get out. The other was confronting the most brutal facts of his situation.

According to Stockdale, those who didn't survive imprisonment were the optimists; the ones who thought they would be out say, at Christmas time. Christmas would come and go and they would still be held captive. Then they would proclaim they would be out by Easter, and once again Easter would come and go and they were still imprisoned.

According to Stockdale, these people eventually died of a broken heart. They had the hope sucked out of them.

Stockdale took a different approach. He opted to confront the most brutal facts of his situation. He steadfastly held onto his belief that he would one day get out but in no way did he deny or ignore the reality that existed around him.

MINDSET SHIFT: *Can you handle the truth?*

I know a woman who has had cancer five times. While her doctors have been able to get her cancer to go into remission, none have actually ever taken the time to help her get her health back.

She mentioned one day that she really wanted to lose weight (she had about fifty pounds to lose) and begin reclaiming her health. I thought about her comment for a few days and decided that I would offer to help (free of charge). I was not claiming to be able to rid her of cancer, but I did think I could pass on what I had learned with my own transformation.

She was totally on board, and the first four weeks she was a model student. She followed all my suggestions along with logging her foods daily. She had dropped about eighteen pounds and lowered her blood pressure as well. She was doing so well, I eased up on checking her daily food logs for a few weeks. When I looked again I noticed that many of her old eating habits had returned.

Fast-food lunches were becoming the norm, and dairy and grains were creeping back into her diet. I sent an e-mail and outlined my observations. I wasn't mean by any stretch, but I gave an honest critique of what needed to be corrected. I ended it by referring back to my own outlook on all this.

My success hinges on getting as much crap (chemicals, sugar, additives, grains) out of my diet as possible. My body affords me little wiggle room. If I want results I need to find ways to eat clean, and I need to challenge traditional thinking (it's not working for about 85% of the population), and I need to challenge my own limits and emotional barriers that prevent me from doing what I know I need to do.

And how did she respond? She no longer speaks to me.

> **THE RIGHT SHI**(F)**T:** *The truth will set you free.*
>
> Brutal honesty is tough. It is painful. It hurts. It makes us sad at times, angry at others. And we often don't want to hear it. But it's also the only thing that paves the way for real change. Without it, all your efforts will lead to deceptive results that won't be sustainable over the long-term.

Opt out of optimism

Inspiration aside, I was intrigued by this concept of acknowledging the brutal facts. When I thought about it within the context of weight-loss, it occurred to me that I had never really been brutally honest with myself.

I began to wonder if I was no different than the POWs who died of a broken heart.

Was I simply an optimist at my core that gave up when my perceived time lines would come and go without the expected results?

I suspected that this could be the brutal truth in regard to my weight-loss goals, so I decided that if I was going to have success moving forward, I was going to have to confront the honest facts of my current situation.

It was a bit humbling to say the least. Below is a list of some things I wrote on January 7, 2011 when I opted to partake in this little exercise.

The bare, brutal facts about me.

⇨ I'm fat.

⇨ I don't like what my body looks like naked (sorry for that visual) or hidden behind strategically bought baggy clothes.

⇨ I'm embarrassed to take my shirt off in public (I'm referring to the beach and not places like a crowded subway or funeral home).

⇨ Being overweight affects my self-confidence in all areas of my life.

⇨ I don't know shit about proper nutrition for my body type.

⇨ I do not have the self-control to have junk food in the house.

⇨ My body is not very forgiving, so my diet must be outstanding!

⇨ I'm an emotional eater.

⇨ When I don't plan my eating, I make bad choices and end up eating crap (not literally, of course).

⇨ I keep waiting for someone else to solve my problems for me.

Beyond my comfort zone...

A few things on that list were hard to write.

The one about my weight affecting my self-confidence wasn't easy. I'm a guy. We're supposed to be too self-confident to admit to low self-confidence, but I knew if I was being truly honest, it affected how I saw myself and therefore affected who I wanted to be in this world.

I also listed that I was an emotional eater. Again, this is something that is usually attributed to women, but guys are as much emotional eaters as women, we are just too stupid (well, at least I am/was) to admit such things.

Others on the list were things I may have thought about briefly but quickly dismissed because I didn't want to confront the truth.

For instance, admitting that I could not have junk food in the house is something I have long thought about but never acted on. I just wasn't prepared to say; "Yeah I have no self-control at this point in my life."

And some of the things were downright eye opening.

Admitting I knew nothing about nutrition was shocking, even for me. I have a degree in Physical and Health Education, so I am no dummy on the topic. But if I was being truthful, it was obvious from my physique that I didn't know that much because I was doing stuff that had kept me fat for twenty-five years.

Confronting the brutal facts was a key evolution to my moving forward because, for the first time, I was embarking on a journey that was not fueled on optimism, but rather on truth.

The goal this time around was to use my brutal facts to obtain results.

FYI: It worked!

MAKE SHI(F)T HAPPEN...

1 You can't **MAKE SHI(F)T HAPPEN** until you are willing to be brutally honest with yourself. You have hidden from yourself long enough. It's time to bring it out into the open and acknowledge what it is so you can begin to make shift happen.

To help, I put together a worksheet and a few guiding questions so you can expose the ten most crucial things you need to acknowledge to begin your transformation.

To get a copy of your own brutally honest worksheet head to . . . www.makeshifthappen.org/resources

YOU CAN'T BE WHO YOU WANT TO BE UNTIL YOU STOP HIDING FROM WHO YOU ARE!

2 Find someone you trust to help you with this next exercise. In the chart below, the scariest quadrant (at least for me) is the one on the bottom right.

What we know about ourselves that others also know.	What we know about ourselves that others <u>don't</u> know.
What we <u>don't</u> know about ourselves that others also <u>don't</u> know.	What we <u>don't</u> know about ourselves that others DO know.

If you are prepared to accept brutal honesty and find out what you don't know about yourself, that fourth quadrant is a goldmine. If you pick the right person, he or she may be able to help you accelerate your growth and transformation by pointing out patterns you weren't even aware of.

WHAT ARE YOUR BLIND SPOTS?

3 This is something many people never address. I have said it before and I'll say it again: brutal honesty is tough, but essential for lasting change. There are reasons why you do what you do, and if you don't address the reasons, then most changes you do implement will be short-lived at best.

If lasting change is your goal then . .

DIG DEEP TO FIND THE REASONS WHY YOU DO WHAT YOU DO!

THE
POWER
OF LESS ⇨

I am like most people. When change is needed, the fix seems to lie in doing *more*.

1. Want to be successful and make more money?
   Then work longer hours

2. Want to create better software?
   Then add more features

3. Want to lose weight?
   Then exercise more

When I embarked on my umpteenth mission to transform my body, I had no clue whether or not this time would be any different than any of the other times I had tried and failed.

But there was one thing I did commit to. If I wanted to get a different result this time around then I needed to commit to being different and doing things differently.

My intuition was that more was MORE, but I had to think counter to what my intuition wanted me to think, because it hadn't helped me reach past weight-loss goals.

What if **MORE** is not the answer?

What if **MORE** is the problem?

What if **MORE** is less?

Feature creep.

I read a book a number of years back called *The Design of Everyday Things*. The author, Donald Norman, was the first person I had encountered who addressed the notion of creeping featurism.

As he put it, *"Creeping featurism is the tendency to add to the number of features that a device can do, often extending the number beyond all reason."*

Somewhere along the way, we have been sold on this perverse idea that MORE is better and I, like many, had unknowingly bought into this.

Take the creep out.

MORE was always my go-to strategy for any and all weight-loss-related issues.

And since that had gotten me nowhere for twenty-five years, I made a decision that my success would lay in doing LESS.

And so I started with . . .

LESS exercise...

Looking back at my exploits in the exercise department, it was pretty darned evident that I suffered from Exercise Creep. My definition:

"Exercise creep is the tendency for those trying to lose weight to add more exercise to their current routine in the hopes of getting slimmer. When that doesn't work, they add more. And when it still doesn't work, they add even more. This reverse pyramid scheme continues until it crumbles under its own weight (no pun intended) and exercise ceases altogether."

Exercise was always the first thing I defaulted to when I was really serious about weight-loss. In fact, as I mentioned back in Shift #20, there was a time where I was working out twice a day. But even then I was thinking, "This isn't realistic. What if I get married? What if I have kids? What if I decide to have a life? What if I stop asking myself "what if" questions?"

So this time around I decided my goal would be **LESS** exercise. Not less in the sense of zero/zilch/nada, but less in the sense of finding the **minimal threshold** I needed to create the changes I wanted. As you shall see in Shift #8: Be 911, exercise is vitally important in my plan to not only ensure my survival, but also the survival of those around me.

LESS time...

One of the smartest innovations I implemented was to distinguish between my **total workout time** and the **actual time** spent doing exercise.

This was hammered home to me one day when some Jesus look-a-like on YouTube talked about getting ready to go for his three-hour workout. I remember thinking, "Really! Three hours! You are doing something seriously wrong if you need to be working out for three hours."

I suspect he was only really exercising for about thirty minutes. The rest of the time would have been spent resting, talking, texting the Apostles, and adjusting his sandals and robe. But that is not working out.

Since knowing that length of time was a critical factor in my level of motivation, I decided that all workouts had to come in at a total time of thirty minutes or less. There was nothing magical about that number other than it felt doable even on a day when my motivation was in the crapper.

While my workout time would be thirty minutes or less, my actual exercise time (excluding rest periods) would range somewhere between ten to twenty minutes, depending on what I was doing and how I was feeling. I have since discovered the average tends to fall in the ten- to fifteen-minute range.

In the beginning, there was a *lot* of trial and error. I would design a tentative workout schedule, determine my intervals (for most timed routines, I do one minute of exercise followed by thirty seconds of rest for twelve to fifteen rounds), and then see if they were doable in the time frame allotted.

Most of the time I got it wrong. We humans tend to overestimate our abilities, and that is exactly what I did on almost each initial program design I created. I would then modify my program and the next week I would try again. It took me about three tries to get my workout routine to come in under thirty minutes.

MINDSHIFT:
The evolution of a workout philosophy

For the first month I was all over the map with my workouts. I was doing all kinds of crazy things, but there was no rhyme or reason to it.

I realized I needed more structure, so I came up with the 5 x 3 Matrix.

Here's how it works. On days when I am doing resistance training, I pick five exercises that allow me to work my entire body (this is key) and perform each exercise for one minute. I rest thirty to sixty seconds in between exercises, depending on how intense I want the workout to be (the less rest, the more intense).

Once I completed all five exercises I would go back and repeat all five in my second and third sets.

If I rested for thirty seconds between exercises, then my total workout would be twenty-two and a half minutes long. If I rested sixty seconds, the total workout would be twenty-nine minutes.

Below is an example of a resistance workout.

Exercise	Set #1	Set #2	Set #3
Pull Ups	15	13	11
Diamond Push Ups	22	19	17
Triceps Dip (UBP)	25	25	23
Sandbag Squat	20	20	20
Sandbag Clean & Press	13	11	12
Total Time	22:30		

THE RIGHT SHI(F)T: *Make it count.*

I am sucking wind when I am done with this workout, and that's the goal when I am doing my resistance training. I need to MAKE IT COUNT! So do you!!

LESS equipment . . .

Equipment is a stumbling block for many, and it's the reason most end up joining a gym.

[Note: I don't recommend joining a gym to anyone trying to lose weight unless they want to remain overweight and out of shape. There is a reason they make you sign a one-year contract. Most never make it out of the first month.]

Lack of equipment is also a great reason to procrastinate and put off starting a program altogether. But truthfully, a great program doesn't require much, which is contrary to what most people believe.

I do all my workouts wherever I happen to be—at home, on vacation, or on a work trip. You can see from the pictures below that I created a kick ass workout at my buddy's cottage (same dude who pointed out my carrot problem) simply using stuff on his property.

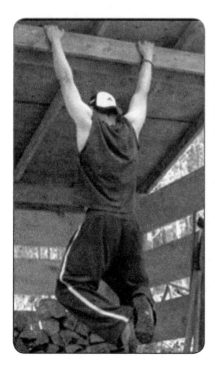 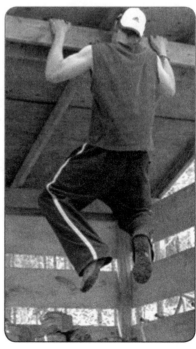

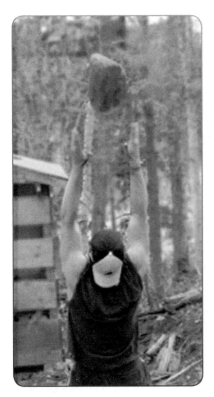 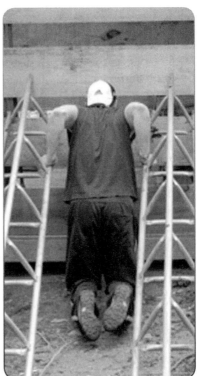

What I like about less equipment is that it really sparks my creativity to seek out and design new exercises and even design my own equipment.

The first picture (top left) is a simple boulder throw (I'm not catching it, even though the picture appears to show otherwise). I would squat and pick up the rock (which weighed about thirty pounds) and then, using both hands, throw it behind me as high and as far as possible.

My pull-ups were done on a recently constructed woodshed, but the dips were the thing I was most proud of (top right). My "dip station" was fashioned from some discarded antennas I found on a neighboring property. I simply leaned them on the open slots of the wood shed and presto, I had a dip station.

I should also point out that I'm not against buying equipment. In fact, it was only recently that I obtained a few pieces I have long wanted. But whatever I buy has to be simple in its design and allow for creative use. By creative use I mean it must enable me to use the piece for at least five different types of exercises.

LESS food . . .

I don't quite mean that as it sounds. I'm not talking about limiting myself to the amount I can eat. I'm actually talking about keeping a very simple grocery list that is comprised of predominantly whole foods.

I'm actually appropriating that idea from Gordon Ramsey and his show *Kitchen Nightmares*. Ever watch an episode? It's actually quite fascinating. In almost all cases, the floundering places he is trying to revive have a vast array of menu choices, most of them lousy.

One of his first changes is chopping the menu down to about ten to twenty items and showing them how to make those dishes superbly.

I have taken that same approach. My grocery list on most weeks has no more than fifteen to twenty items on it.

What I like about this is that I tend to spend less (which I found very surprising), I'm much more creative in the kitchen (creative means I actually use the garlic I bought), and virtually no food spoils.

LESS money . . .

It's always easy to throw money at a problem, but I think the most effective solutions come from bootstrapping.

I have vowed *not* to throw money at this problem, opting for creativity instead.

I have no gym membership. For the first eight months I did not purchase a single piece of exercise equipment. I used equipment I had for years that was simply collecting dust. My grocery bill is less mostly because I do not purchase any expensive supplements that the "experts" say you must have.

LESS has mostly certainly proven to be MORE in my case.

MAKE SHI(F)T HAPPEN...

1 Try to wrap your head around the idea that LESS can be MORE. As I mentioned above, it was a weird notion for me to embrace, but I now see the brilliance in this simple approach.

Less is also more sustainable over the long run. More is not. Seek to find your minimal threshold in all aspects of this journey.

EMBRACE THE MINDSET LESS CAN BE MORE!

---

2 Embrace the idea of keeping workouts to thirty minutes or less. The key to the workout is intensity, not duration. I have found that ten to fifteen minutes of intense resistance training is far superior to mindless half-ass workouts that border on sixty minutes or more. Just remember: when it is time to work out . . .

MAKE IT COUNT!

---

3 Try out the 5 x 3 matrix with the idea of making it uniquely yours. Adopt a few of my ideas to start out and then look to create a program over time that works specifically for your needs.

To get a blank 5 x 3 worksheet that you can customize to suit your needs go to . . .
www.makeshifthappen.org/resources

You will also find a few sample workouts you can steal as well.

STEAL IDEAS SHAMELESSLY!

BE 911 ⇨

had always thought my exercise program was a tool for weight-loss. Consequently, everything I did was in the name of shedding pounds, whether I was slogging away on a stationary bike, taking part in some kind of extreme cardio session, or biking my ass off around the city of Toronto.

But I had finally accumulated enough evidence to realize that exercise in and of itself had very little impact on my fat loss. Using the twenty-five years of data I collected (also known as my big fat body), it was clear I needed to redefine my philosophy.

So I started with this . . .

My Fat Loss Is 100 Percent Diet Related.

This declaration completely shifted my focus. I was not saying exercise didn't have an impact on fat loss, but I realized it played a very small role in the whole process, especially early on.

In fact, I believe the relationship between diet and exercise shifts as we transform from fat and out-of-shape couch potatoes to lean, active go-getters.

Impact of Diet and Exercise on Fat Loss

Stage #	Stage Name	Diet	Exercise
1	Fat and out of shape	99%+	<1%
2	Early stages of weight-loss	95%	5%
3	Middle stages of weight-loss	90%	10%
4	Late stages of weight-loss	85%	15%
5	State of leanness achieved	80%	20%

Now that I finally understood how important diet was to my fat loss, I needed to shift my view on my exercise program. I needed to reframe it to more accurately reflect what it was intended to do for me.

And then I came across this quote . . .

> *"Every man should be able to save his own life. He should be able to swim far enough, run fast and long enough to save his life in case of emergency and necessity. He also should be able to chin himself a reasonable number of times, as well as to dip a number of times, and he should be able to jump a reasonable height and distance."*

> —*Earle E. Liederman, Endurance*

Liederman wrote this in his book *Endurance* back in 1926. It is still extremely relevant, although it is seldom practiced in its literal sense today.

But this quote fascinated me and instantly challenged my perception of what an exercise program could and should do for me.

INITIAL ASSESSMENT: *What can you do?*

Based on Liederman's notion of survival, complete the chart below to get a baseline of where your abilities currently lie.

Exercise	1st Attempt	2nd Attempt (1 month later)
Push Ups (to exhaustion)		
Pull ups (to exhaustion)		
Dips (to exhaustion)		
100 meter sprint (time)		
1km Swim (time)		
Vertical Leap (inches)		

Don't worry about where your numbers are initially. But include these exercises in your training and test on a monthly basis to assess your progress.

The profile of a survivor . . .

It also brought me back to an idea that I thought about often after reading a fascinating book called, *The Unthinkable: Who Survives When Disaster Strikes—and Why* by Amanda Ripley.

Ripley mentioned that survival, on its most basic of levels, becomes a matter of physics. The heavier someone is, the lower their physical abilities. So things like running, climbing over objects, or being able to pull one's own body weight are greatly hampered. That doesn't leave someone with many options when an emergency or disaster strikes.

Ripley also cited studies that showed that obese people are three times more likely to die in car crashes, partly because their health makes it difficult to recover from injury.

Follow-up studies from 9/11 also showed that obese people were three times more likely to be hurt or injured.

As sad as this was, I couldn't help but wonder how many people died in the 9/11 attacks because their health prevented them from getting to safety. And while no one has ever publicly stated this, it would be logical to assume that certain people with poor health prevented healthy people from getting out safely as well.

This was the first time in my life that I realized the effects of poor health extended far beyond the individual. My poor health didn't just affect me. It could in fact cause others injury or even death.

I was determined to make sure that would never be the case.

Could I survive?

Sometimes I wonder how I would have fared if I have been present during the massive Tsunami that hit Indonesia on December 26, 2004.

I have imagined myself standing on that beach and seeing that massive wave rolling in. Beside me is a three-year-old little girl playing in the sand.

Like many of those that were there that day, I have no doubt that I would not have realized what was happening until the very last minute.

What would I have needed to do to survive? To help others survive?

In order to have any chance, I would have had to grab the little girl and literally throw her over my shoulder and then sprint for a sustained period of time as fast as I could to higher ground. That might have meant bounding up the stairs of a nearby hotel (which many survivors did in fact do), all with an added 30 pounds on my shoulder.

Would I have been physically capable of doing this? Could I have saved that little girl and myself?

Honestly, I am not so sure.

These are not pleasant questions or thoughts to have, but they are realistic, and it caused me to radically reevaluate what I wanted my body to be able to do.

(Note: the odds of being in a disaster are slim, but that doesn't mean much if the odds work against you even one time.)

Being 911...

It also got me thinking about a variety of worst-case scenarios. Forget about calling 911 in an emergency! Could I be 911 in those situations?

⇨ Did I have the endurance to swim a kilometer or more if a boat capsized?

⇨ Could I swim out to save a drowning victim?

⇨ Could I carry someone weighing 180 pounds out of a burning house?

⇨ Could I pull someone to safety in a car crash if there was fear of a gas explosion?

⇨ Did I have the speed and agility to get to a child who was about to run into a busy street?

⇨ Could I pull my own body weight if I needed to pull myself to safety in the case of a flood or to avoid an animal attack of some kind?

⇨ Could I pull someone else up to safety?

I must admit I didn't like the answers to those questions. I could barely do a pull up. I had not sprinted in any capacity in about fifteen years, and I doubted I could save that drowning victim or get to that child who was about to dart into oncoming traffic.

There are thousands upon thousands of people every year who have to live with that reality. I didn't want to be one of those statistics.

I also understood that my body was something I had complete control over and decided that I needed to redesign my exercise program to accommodate the situations listed above.

Survivorman...

And that is when I decided that my exercise program would be geared entirely for my survival.

With this idea now firmly planted in my brain, a subtle shift took place.

If my program was going to be used for survival, it needed to be functional. It needed to allow me to do stuff I couldn't currently do.

My program needed to focus on building strength and speed that would translate to real-world scenarios. Riding a stationary bike while watching the evening news applies to zippo in the real world.

I completely redesigned my workouts and started adding things that I had either avoided or never done because they were just too much work.

Survival (or ensuring the survival of others) dictated I add the following:

⇨ all variety of pull ups

⇨ push ups of all kinds

⇨ dead lifts

⇨ squats

⇨ sprinting, stairs and other forms of speed work

⇨ swimming (sprints in the pool)

⇨ total body exercises (that focus on multiple muscle groups)

⇨ exercises that involve everyday objects like large water jugs, barrels, rocks, etc.

⇨ extreme strength-building exercises

⇨ jumping

⇨ agility-type exercises

It also dictated that I subtract the following:

⇨ isolation exercises for vanity reasons only

⇨ cardio without purpose

⇨ a toning approach (toning is not functional in the real world)

This shift in my exercise mission statement has had many wonderful side effects.

It has allowed me to bring excitement and creativity to my workouts. I have been able to push the boundaries of what my body is able to do. I'm closing in on seventeen pull-ups when I could only do two at the beginning. My weekly sprint workout rocks (even though I look like Kermit the Frog when I run).

And I love the idea of pushing my body's capabilities, whether with the goal of being able to do a one-armed pull-up (which I can now do) or running fifty meters with a 100-pound-weight over my shoulder.

MAKE SHI(F)T HAPPEN...

1 Could you save your own life if disaster struck? Could you save the life of someone else? Your child? Your spouse? A stranger? Don't take this lightly. Think about the implications of this, and if your answer is "No" (and it is for most people), commit to taking action *now* to rectify this.

IN AN EMERGENCY, COULD YOU SAVE A LIFE? COULD YOU BE 911?

2 Take some time to do the **Initial Assessment**. Below are a few suggestions on how to accomplish it using some of the free resources that are available.

1. Find a track in your area, and after doing an appropriate warm-up, run 100 meters and record your time.

2. Hit the local pool and find out how long it would take you to swim one kilometer.

3. Hit the local playground and use the monkey bars to find out how many pull-ups you can do.

4. Then head home and use two sturdy chairs to see how many dips you can do.

5. Then drop down and see how many push-ups you can do.

6. Last, stand by a wall and extend one arm up as high as you can and with a pencil mark the area. Then jump up as high as you can and use the pencil (chalk is better) to mark you height. Measure the distance between points to get your vertical jump.

ONLY WHEN YOU KNOW WHERE YOU STARTED CAN YOU KNOW WHERE YOU ARE GOING!

3 Take ownership of your own program. By this I mean look to create something that works for you as opposed to relying on someone else to create something for you. Use the four components of a highly successful body (see Shift #6) to help guide you in creating something that increases the functionality of your body.

DON'T RELY ON OTHERS TO SOLVE YOUR PROBLEM!

SMASH THE SCALE ⇨

There is nothing more demoralizing than having a week where you have eaten super-clean and have had rock-solid workouts only to plop yourself down on the scale and discover you have lost no weight at all or . . . gasp! . . . that you actually put on a few pounds.

If you're like me, you have had that scenario play out numerous times. It's frustrating to say the least, but when I began putting the ideas of my new approach together, I knew I needed to address this issue, otherwise my psyche was going to get beat down like a dirty rug. And I knew this would probably cause me to quit (again) if this was the sole measure of my progress.

Why the scale is a flawed measure of success . . .

At a party recently a friend asked me how much I weighed. I laughed and said I had no idea, which drew a look of surprise. The truth is I have not weighed myself in about a decade. In fact, it might even be longer than that.

I gave up on the scale as a measurement of my progress for many reasons. The biggest being that I believe it is a flawed measure of success. It does not factor in any of the really important stuff like the increased functionality of my body (i.e., going from two pull-ups to seventeen), it does not factor in my newfound discipline (I am only eating three treats per week), it does not ensure that I will achieve the look I desire and, most important, it does not guarantee that I will be happy with the end result.

MINDSHIFT: *Smash the scale... literally*

A client of mine, Trudy, shared her story about the scale after we had been working together for about a month.

I take a very different approach than most who help people change how they look. While diet and exercise play a role, I get my clients to focus on a total of eight to ten VITAL BEHAVIORS. When these behaviors are fixed, and remain fixed, it can lead to startling personal transformation.

In our first month, Trudy had done an amazing job focusing on the KEY BEHAVIORS that encourage weight-loss. She recorded what she ate daily, she cut out key foods that made her fat, and she started introducing short stints of resistance training two or three times a week.

Her results immediately started to appear. She lost twenty-one total inches (this was after the first six weeks) and, more importantly, for the first time in her life she *knew* she was going to achieve something that had eluded her for most of her adult life: a body she could be proud of.

The best part is, she *did not* use a scale to track her progress. In fact, she owned a glass scale and literally hammered the shit out of it and threw it in the garbage. She was tired of focusing on a number that constantly left her feeling deflated and defeated.

She has now found a much healthier set of indicators to measure her progress. Among those, she takes her body measurements regularly and uses the feedback from how her clothes fit to judge the progress she is making.

On a recent call she told me that a new skirt she had made specifically to her measurements just before we started working together no longer fit. In fact, it almost fell off while she was riding public transit.

That's a problem she's happy to have!

THE RIGHT SHI(F)T: *Say "happy trails" to the scale*

Get rid of your scale. Smash it, blend it, or drop it off a high building. However you dispose of it, just know there are far better indicators out there that will help you gauge your success.

I was going for a new look, and that "look" would weigh whatever it was supposed to weigh; it might be 150 pounds, hell, it might even be 180 pounds! I DIDN'T CARE. Nor did I care to be stereotyped by all those ridiculous body mass index charts that many people are judged by.

You know those charts. The ones where people of a certain height should be a certain weight. It's not the dumbest thing ever created (don't get me started on IQ tests), but it's pretty darn close.

I'm not sure what your experience is, but I have seen what these charts do to people. They make people feel awful about themselves when they don't fit into this accepted "norm."

How will I know?

I resolved that I would continue on the path of *never* weighing myself. The question now was, "How will I know when I have reached the look I want to achieve?"

For that, I decided to borrow an idea from Mohammed Yunus.

Banker to the Poor . . .

Mohammed Yunus is credited with being the pioneer behind the microcredit movement. He is also the bestselling author of the book *Banker to the Poor* and runs Grameen Bank, a bank dedicated to issuing microloans to help the poor pull themselves out of poverty.

He has created some truly remarkable change, and if you get a chance, I highly recommend reading his book. It is extremely inspirational.

How to know when someone has dug themselves out of poverty?

This was a question Yunus and his team had struggled with. If they were going to run a successful, results-driven business helping the poor get out of poverty, then they needed a set of indicators that would demonstrate success.

These indicators would also have to be taught to the poor, so that they had a measuring stick to know when they had pulled themselves out of poverty.

ECONOMIC SHIFT: *You are no longer poor if…*

Here are the ten criteria Yunus and his staff developed that would help identify when a member and his or her family moved out of poverty:

1. The family lives in a house worth at least Tk. 25,000 (US$330) or a house with a tin roof, and each member of the family is able to sleep on a bed instead of on the floor.
   (The taka is the currency for Bangladesh.)

2. Family members drink pure water from tube-wells, boiled water, or water purified by using alum, arsenic-free, purifying tablets or pitcher filters.

3. All children in the family over six years of age are all going to school or have finished primary school.

4. Minimum weekly loan installment of the borrower is Tk. 200 or more.

5. Family uses sanitary latrine.

6. Family members have adequate clothing for everyday use, warm clothing for winter, such as shawls, sweaters, blankets, etc, and mosquito nets to protect themselves from mosquitoes.

7. Family has sources of additional income, such as a vegetable garden or fruit-bearing trees, so that they are able to fall back on these sources of income when they need additional money.

8. The borrower maintains an average annual balance of Tk. 5,000 in her savings accounts.

9. Family experiences no difficulty in having three square meals a day throughout the year (i.e., no member of the family goes hungry any time of the year).

10. Family can take care of health. If any member of the family falls ill, they can afford to take all necessary steps to seek adequate healthcare.

I absolutely love this model because it is all-encompassing and more accurately reflects a quality of life that can't be captured by simply saying people needed to achieve "X" dollars per year.

This is why the measurement of weight fails so badly. That number on the scale just doesn't capture any of the acquired intangibles or the improved quality of life that comes with a newly created body.

My twelve core indicators . . .

So I set about coming up with my own indicators to know when I had created not only the body I wanted, but also the confidence and peace of mind that comes with such an achievement.

As I have traveled further into this personal odyssey, I have come to understand that this is as much a journey into self-acceptance as it is a journey to transform my body.

My indicators accurately reflect my evolution on this matter.

1. I never need to know how much I weigh to feel great about how I look.

2. I'm comfortable naked (once again, I apologize for that mental image). When I stand in front of a mirror, I like how I look.

3. I have no visible body fat on any part of my body; there is noticeable muscle separation; I can see my abs.

4. I can see veins in my forearms, calves, and lower abdominal wall (a clear indicator of fat loss).

5. The waist size on my pants is between 28 to 30 inches.

6. I consistently work out four to six times each week without fail.

7. I record everything I eat everyday without exception, along with notes and ideas of what is and isn't working.

8. I am able to successfully assess problems, come up with appropriate solutions, and get back on track immediately.

9. My diet is 90 percent paleo, week in and week out.

10. The whole approach is sustainable one year, five years, even ten years from now.

11. I know with absolute certainty that what I am doing is right and that I will never resort back to my old ways.

12. I can do the following with my body:

    ⇨ Run 100 meters in under 16 seconds

    ⇨ Do 15–20 pull-ups (without coming off bar)

    ⇨ Do 40–50 push-ups (nonstop)

    ⇨ Do 25+ dips (nonstop)

    ⇨ Carry 100 pounds on my shoulder for 50 meters

    ⇨ Jump up onto something waist high from a standing position

    ⇨ Climb a 15-foot rope

MAKE SHI(F)T HAPPEN...

1 Get rid of your scale. Seriously, that stupid thing just wreaks havoc with your mind. Few have the ability to see that number simply as feedback. Most tend to personalize the results, and it ends up ruining what might well have been a great day. If this is you I am describing, then I suggest the following . . .

TREAT YOUR SCALE LIKE A SALAD & TOSS IT!

---

2 Create your own unique set of indicators to know when you have achieved your desired look. As I have suggested throughout this book, borrow liberally from my stuff as well as any of the other ideas I have presented. Just remember to create something that is uniquely you.

For a complete copy of mine, go to . .
www.makeshifthappen.org/resources

TO MAKE PROGRESS, YOU MUST FIRST KNOW HOW TO MEASURE IT!

---

3 Do yourself a favor and get a copy of *Banker to the Poor*. Not only is it an amazingly inspirational story, but if you keep a lookout, you will also find many ideas that you can use within the context of your own life.

LOOK TO APPROPIATE PRINCIPLES IN UNRELATED AREAS AND APPLY THEM TO YOUR JOURNEY!

4 COMPONENTS OF A HIGHLY SUCCESSFUL BODY ⇨

I mentioned back in Shift #8 that I do not equate fat loss with exercise. Some may mistake that as meaning I don't think exercise is important. On the contrary, I think exercise is extremely important, but I'm not looking at it through the lens of fat loss. I look at through the lens of survival and quality of life.

Study the elderly . . .

Do you want to know what you will become when you get older? Go to a mall and spend some time watching the elderly.

Be forewarned, it won't be pretty. That's why people fear growing old.

Vast majorities of the elderly have done little to take care of themselves (it's not entirely their fault, as they came from a generation in which exercise wasn't a priority). As a result, many suffer from limited mobility and experience difficulty simply supporting their own body weight.

In most cases you will find that these individuals have done nothing to enhance the four main components of a healthy body.

Redefining Exercise . . .

I *do not* want to become that person who suffers immeasurably in his later years because I neglected myself in the first half of my life. I don't want to be seventy years old and forced to walk with a cane, or worse, confined to one of those scooters because I opted not to take care of myself now.

While I acknowledge that luck does factor in to whether or not you are hindered by crippling illness, disease, or accidents, I also believe you create your own luck by managing those things you have direct control over, such as:

⇨ what you put in your body

⇨ how you use your body

⇨ how you use your mind to influence your actions

The four components
of a highly successful body . . .

Have you ever read Stephen Covey's *The Seven Habits of Highly Successful People*? It's sold like twenty million copies, so chances are you at least know the basic premise behind the book.

If not, let me give you the Deano Cliff Notes:
> *Time management is best accomplished when we organize our tasks and activities (goals) around the various roles in our life.*

I love the concept because it implies that time management is dynamic and interactive within the context of our lives, not some static irrelevant to-do list where we simply check off completed tasks each day to show how productive we've been.

It occurred to me that this same principle could apply to my body as well. It seemed logical that our body also has roles. By roles I mean functional components that need to be optimized to maintain maximum efficiency.

I donned my thinking cap (OK, it's a shower cap), put my degree in Physical and Health Education to work, and determined there are really four roles of a highly successful body.

They are . . .

Strength	lift heavy things; push & pull one's own body weight numerous times
Endurance	go far at a steady pace
Speed/Agility	go as fast as you can (be shifty)
Flexibility	maximize movement around all joint areas (be bendy)

I prefer to look at the four in the context of a quadrant. As you can see from the diagram on the next page, each component is assigned its own quadrant, and each quadrant is divided into three sections, numbered 1, 2, or 3.

Four Components of a Highly Successful Body

Strength Examples
Weight training
Body weight exercises
Rock climbing

Speed Examples
Sprints: Flat surface, hills, stairs
Plyometrics: Jump training
Biking: Outdoors, spin class,
Swimming

1. Strength

Lift heavy things
Push & pull
body
weight
2
3
1

2. Speed

Go as fast
as you
can
!!!
2
3
1

3. Flexibility

Maximize range
of motion
of joints
2
3
1

4. Endurance

Go far at
a steady
pace
2
3
1

Flexibility Examples
Yoga, Stretching, Pilates,
Martial Arts

Endurance Examples
Walking, Biking, Hiking,
Running, Sports

* each number represents 30 minutes total time.

The goal of any complete workout program is much the same as Covey's insight: each week we need to ensure that we spend sufficient time in each quadrant. The example above illustrates the number of workout sessions I expect to accomplish in each quadrant. In any particular week, I will have two strength workouts (quadrant 1), one speed workout (quadrant 2), one flexibility workout (quadrant 3), and two or three endurance-training sessions (quadrant 4). By the end of the week, I have managed to hit each quadrant, ensuring that I am nurturing a well-balanced physique.

BULLSHI(F)T: *A BIG mistake many make*

Many people have no real plan when they are looking to lose weight other than a vague notion they need to do something. Consequently, they often make the mistake of spending their time in only one quadrant.

For example, there are many people who walk. Walking is great, but that cannot be your entire workout, as it hits the endurance quadrant only.

The same goes for those who hit the weights. Weight training done correctly works on strength building, but that cannot be all that you do.

I have seen more than my share of fat, flabby runners. While I think most should not be running at all, it does meet the endurance requirements. But again, that *cannot* be all that you do.

Yoga is great for working on the much-neglected flexibility component, but that cannot be all that you do.

THE RIGHT SHI(F)T: *Increase the number of quadrants, not hours.*

Begin to look for ways to expand the number of quadrants in which you spend your time. The more quadrants you explore, the more functional your body becomes.

Troubleshooting . . .

The problem, however, is that most people don't really think about the "componentry" of their body, so if they train at all (big IF), they tend to focus on one, maybe two quadrants at most.

To give this some context, let's go back to Covey's concept.

Imagine you have identified the following roles in your life:

⇨ father or mother

⇨ husband or wife

⇨ son or daughter

⇨ boss/owner or employee

What would happen if you neglected two of these areas altogether? By neglect I mean you spent no time (0 minutes) attending to that quadrant.

For instance, what if you neglected the role of husband or wife entirely? How successful do you think your marriage would be?

You get the point here.

So when we are looking at transforming our bodies, we need to be aware that neglect in one quadrant can lead to serious health repercussions down the road.

And while the goal is to ensure you are hitting each quadrant at least once each week (more if possible, depending on the role), it is equally important to ensure that the activity you partake in has value and fits into a master plan.

Let's go back to the husband or wife role for a moment. There is a huge difference between a weekly date night where it is just the two of you as opposed to, say, going to a friend's party together. The quality of the first activity is infinitely more valuable than the second based on the quality of one-on-one time that a date night creates. It's possible to spend zero time together at a party.

So too it is with the body and exercise.

It's important to be in each quadrant at least once each week.

And it is equally important to partake in high-value activities. Riding a stationary bike while reading the newspaper is an excellent example of a low-value task that gives the appearance of work done but does little to generate quality results down the road.

A program with purpose . . .

Having a purpose behind the program has had an IMMENSE impact on my success. It's the first time in my life that I actually had a working philosophy about my health that went beyond vague and general ideas like "get healthy" and "lose weight."

Honestly, in the past I simply did stuff so I could say I was doing stuff. But there was no rhyme or reason to my actions.

This might also explain why I could never maintain these programs for any length of time. They didn't fit into a larger vision or master plan.

This model changes all of that. My program now takes on a chess-like demeanor. Exercises are like pieces on the board. Each has a role. Each serves a purpose. Each can do a different thing. And each must be strategically played to ensure the best results.

And each time I start a new game (learn something new that allows me to add to or update my database of exercises), I move closer to mastery.

MAKE SHI(F)T HAPPEN...

1 Embrace the notion that your body has different roles much like you have different roles in your life. Each role is important to a well-rounded body. Take the next thirty days to create a workout program for yourself that has you spending time in each quadrant at least once a week.

COMMIT TIME EACH WEEK TO EACH COMPONENT OF A HIGHLY SUCCESSFUL BODY!

---

2 Print off two copies of "The four components of a highly successful body" diagram. Post one copy where you will see it often to help remind you of the balance you are striving for.

Use the second to sketch out ideas of exercises and activities you could partake in to help you to achieve that balance.

To download your own copy, go to . . .
www.makeshifthappen.org/resources

DESIGN SOMETHING FOR EACH QUADRANT THAT IS UNIQUELY YOU!

---

3 Find innovative ways to motivate yourself to complete your workouts. Try using your online calendar (I use iCal) to schedule your workouts for the week. Pick a time and day for each, and in brackets include the quadrant it hits.

Be sure to choose a time when you have energy as opposed to a time where you will be running on fumes. When you schedule exercise poorly, it is much easier to skip a workout.

HONOR YOUR WORKOUT APPOINTMENTS LIKE YOU WOULD A BUSINESS MEETING!

RECOVER LIKE WILE E. COYOTE ⇨

For twenty-five years I made the same stupid mistakes over and over again when I was attempting to transform my body.

Mistake #1...

I always defaulted to exercise in an attempt to lose weight. For some reason, I had it in my thick skull that I wasn't doing enough, no matter how much I had done previously.

Invariably I would design a program that focused on the concept of more: more exercise, more time, and more days working out. Unfortunately, my approach was extremely shortsighted and completely unrealistic in its expectations.

In hindsight, the only thing MORE achieved was setting myself up for MORE failure.

Mistake #2...

Next, I would attack my diet. I would do the same lamebrain thing each and every time.

I was going to eat healthy.

There are a plethora of reasons why this is just dumb. For starters, the word "healthy" is just way too vague. It is subjective in nature and open for debate. What is healthy for one person can be a fast track to obesity for someone else.

The word "healthy" is also outcome based. Consequently, it lacks any mention of specific behaviors to adopt and measure. So when failure occurs (and I promise you it will) there are no specifics that you can analyze and tweak.

BULLSHI(F)**T:** *Go bananas for bananas*

When I was a vegetarian/vegan, I would eat more bananas in a typical day than most monkeys.

I would include them in my two daily smoothies (bananas not monkeys) and use them for snacks as well. I was easily eating two to four bananas per day.

It was not until I adopted the paleo lifestyle that I discovered that bananas were killing my physique, even though they are considered a "healthy" food.

And here is why they are not a healthy food for me. One banana has about 35g of carbs. That's a lot of carbs. Add that to everything else I was eating and I was over-CARB-onating my body.

I will expand on this in more detail in Shift #2 when I talk about discovering your carb threshold, but I now limit my banana consumption to two or three a week.

THE RIGHT SHI(F)**T:**
Leave the bananas for the monkeys

Not all "health" foods are created equal. What may work for one body may not work for yours. Become the expert on you. Begin to test what actually works for your body type and what doesn't.

Mistake #3...

My inner food fascist would make a blanket proclamation, "No junk food for you!"

This proclamation seemed like a good thing, but what it really did was agitate my inner food rebel. I might be able to curb the rebel activities for a time, but gradually they would wear down my resolve and the junk food cravings would take over.

Anatomy of a meltdown...

Each and every time I would launch into a new lifestyle, the following occurred:

For two or three weeks I was a freaking superstar. I would be:

➡ Eating "healthy"

➡ Doing my insanely unforgiving workout routine

➡ Denying my body the junk food it called out for every damn day

But then, without notice, the meltdown sequence would be activated. Later I discovered that it could be launched by any one of the following:

➡ A shitty day at work

➡ Frustration with lifestyle choices (or lack thereof)

➡ Money concerns

➡ Exhaustion

➡ Lack of results in the area of body transformation

➡ Guilt

➡ Sadness

➡ Stress

➡ Women (and if I was a woman I would most assuredly say men)

When one of these activated the meltdown sequence, all hell broke loose.

First, I would miss a workout. Simultaneously, the missing of a workout would deactivate the food fascist. The coast was now clear to eat junk food.

Or so I thought.

The food fascist's sidekick, Guilt, was actually lurking in the bushes, and when I lapsed he would appear with his little soapbox in tow to lecture me about the virtues of discipline, perseverance, and determination. To add salt to my wounds, he would issue me a citation for failure to appear at a scheduled workout. Damn it! Then he would issue me another for possession of junk food contraband. Double damn it!

Two citations in one day would weigh heavily on me. So much so that I would tempt guilt again the next day to see if I could somehow game the system and fly under his radar. Again guilt would appear, and again I would come away with two more citations. Quadruple damn it!

It was at this point that I would begin to spiral out of control, and before long I was back to doing the same fat-inducing behaviors I had always done.

Understanding monumental change...

It took me twenty-five years to learn.

When you attempt to do something that is so monumental in nature that you need to make Everest-sized changes to your life, you most certainly will fail to reach the summit.

Small adjustments and changes are a much better way to get you from base camp to base camp until you've reached your goals. Small, manageable modifications not only disrupt your life less, but they also help measure success incrementally. If you make a small change and fail, you know what caused you to fail and you can correct it.

Make no mistake: you should be experiencing failure. You will have days where you eat like a rabid hyena. You will have days where workouts are skipped. You will have days (many of them, in fact) where it seems nothing is working and your results have hit a plateau.

That is to be expected.

MINDSHIFT: *Stuck at 301 pounds*

I interviewed Jimmy Moore, who is the host of the very popular *Livin' La Vida Low Carb* show and blog.

Jimmy has an interesting story. He used to weigh just over 400 pounds. He finally got to a point in his life where he'd had enough of the guilt and shame that came with being so extremely overweight.

He did some poking around and eventually adopted a low-carb diet.

(Note: He has since adopted the paleo diet, which has some overlapping principles with the low-carb movement.)

Within 100 days he had lost over 100 pounds and was down around 301 pounds. Then the unthinkable happened. He did not lose a single pound for the next ten weeks. He could not break the 300-pound barrier.

But he soldiered on like he had done for the previous twelve weeks. Why? Because he truly believed the new behaviors he had adopted were worth continuing, even if the results weren't coming as fast or as easily as they once were.

The result? Well, he did eventually break through that barrier and went on to lose an additional 70+ pounds.

THE RIGHT SHI(F)T: *Don't let temporary failure derail you*

When you shift from outcome-based results (i.e., I want to lose 30 pounds) to adopting vital behaviors that set the stage for long-term health and wellness, you are able to weather the storm when you hit a plateau.

To learn more about Jimmy and the great work he is doing, head over to www.livinlavidalowcarb.com.

To watch my interview with him in its entirety, check out www.makeshifthappen.org/resources.

Recover like Wile E. Coyote...

Realizing failure is a precursor to success, I needed to have a recovery plan in place so when it did arrive I could quickly get back on track and continue moving forward on my quest.

And that was when Wile E. Coyote popped into my head.

I used to watch Bugs Bunny all the time as a kid. Each show had a segment where Wile E. Coyote was out to catch the Roadrunner.

No matter how cunning Wile was, he always managed to blow himself up, fall off a cliff, get crushed by a massive boulder, or get flattened by a transport trailer.

And yet, in the next scene, there was Wile, battered and bruised and occasionally flat as a pancake, but right back at his attempts to capture that pesky roadrunner.

Here is the lesson we can all learn from our animated little friend.

When failure occurs, you need to recover quickly. Don't wallow in it. Understand that it is part of the process. It is going to happen. It's supposed to happen. So you deal with it.

BUT here is the key. You need to have a plan in place to clean up the mess and get back on track.

How to recover when you fail

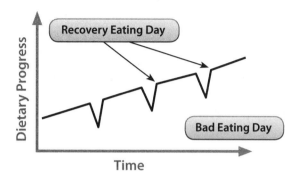

A recovery day...

When I have an eating day where I have gone off course (my euphemism for "I ate a bunch of crap I should not have"), I go into recovery mode.

First, if my day is not complete, I make sure my next meal and all remaining meals are in line with the philosophy I have created for myself. This is really important. I need to interrupt the pattern immediately.

The brilliance of this little maneuver is it helps me squash guilt. I'm as good as my last meal, so if I make the follow-up super-clean, then I am right back on track.

Second, I immediately go to my recovery-eating day that I have already mapped out in advance for just such occasions. The key here is this is a day that I have designed before failure has ever occurred. I don't wait until it happens to decide what (if anything) I am going to do. I know what to do when that day comes.

Here is what that day looks like:

Meal #1: Three eggs, coconut oil, spinach, dandelion, and zucchini with raw tomato and avocado

Snack #1: ¼ cup of raw almonds

Meal #2: Monster tuna salad (all raw veggies with homemade oil and balsamic vinegar dressing)

Snack #2: ¼ cup of raw almonds

Meal #3: Homemade chicken soup with steamed veggies and butter

Snack #3: ¾ cup of frozen blueberries with cinnamon

Macronutrient Breakdown...

Food Summary				
Meal	Calories	Fat	Carbs	Protein
Breakfast	484	35.4g	18.7g	23.9g
Snack #1	252	21.0g	8.4g	8.4g
Lunch	344	14.2g	17.2g	40.9g
Snack #2	252	21.0g	8.4g	8.4g
Dinner	280	15.2g	20.5g	20.5g
Snack #3	82	0.5g	21.0g	1.1g
Total	**1694**	107.3g	94.2g	103.2g
Percentage of Calories [1]		55%	21%	24%

There are a few things to notice above.

First, I *don't* starve myself. That is not the solution. The goal is to have a super-clean eating day that comes in under 100grams of carbs. I talk more about this in Shift #2: Discover Your Carb Threshold.

Second, I strive for a calorie count that is somewhere between 1,700 and 2,000 calories. That range seems to be optimal when I am looking to "lean-out."

In case you are wondering, I determined that amount based on the data I collected over the past eight months by using my food diary. Again, I cannot stress enough the importance of food logging and creating a meal plan designed for your body type.

MAKE SHI(F)T HAPPEN...

1 Decide in advance what your recovery mode eating day is going to look like. Use mine as an example, but create something that is geared to your particular body type. Be sure to plug it into the program you are using to log your foods and then print it off and post it somewhere that is easily accessible.

DECIDE HOW TO RESPOND TO FAILURE IN ADVANCE!

2 Extend this idea to other areas where failure will most certainly occur. For instance, decide in advance how you are going to deal with a missed workout or an unexpected appointment that might drastically reduce the time available for a workout.

A TEN-MINUTE WORKOUT IS BETTER THAN NO WORKOUT AT ALL!

3 Commit to changing how you think. Focus on changing *behaviors* rather than relying on outcomes. Outcome-based goals are impossible to recover from because they have no identifiable behavior attached that can be changed.

FOCUS ON VITAL BEHAVIORS THAT ARE SUSTAINABLE AND ENCOURAGE LONG-TERM HEALTH!

ABORT!
SYSTEM
FAILURE ⇨

If you haven't had a chance to read *Switch* by Chip and Dan Heath, then this is another book I would highly recommend. It is chock full of advice on how to make change happen.

And don't mistake this for a business book either. They talk about principles that can be applied to numerous situations, whether it is raising children or altering one's leadership style.

One of the concepts they introduced was something called the Fundamental Attribution Error (FAE). It can best be defined this way:

People tend to ignore the situational forces that shape other people's behavior, thus attributing it to the way they are rather than the situation they are in.

A great example to illustrate this is with the ever-popular ATM machines. Not all that long ago the process went like this:

1. Insert bank card and enter pin number

2. Choose account and enter amount of cash to withdraw

3. Remove cash that is dispensed

4. Remove bankcard

Nothing seems amiss here, but banks were dealing with a high volume of complaints as an inordinate number of people were leaving without removing their bankcard.

Now it might be easy to call these people idiots (a bit harsh I think), or the much nicer but also not complimentary "absent-minded." But if you were to set up a video camera and watch more closely, what you would notice is that there is something within the situation that creates the absent-mindedness. Do you know what it is?

If you are not sure, here is a hint. What is the first thing you do when you take your money out of the machine? You count it (or, in my case, I like to fall to my knees and raise my hands in the air and yell, "I WON!"). The simple act of counting was enough to cause a great many people to walk away, completely forgetting to take their card.

With a complete understanding of the problem, the solution becomes quite obvious. Tweak the situation (the process) by simply switching around steps 3 and 4. This eliminates the problem altogether, as it would be highly unlikely people are going to walk away without taking their money.

BULLSHI(F)**T:** *An exception to every rule*

On two occasions in my life, I have walked away from a cash machine without taking my money. Both times I withdrew $80, and both times I forgot to take it.

The first time I completely forgot to remove my money because I was on the phone with my bank talking about a credit card issue. Seems ironic, doesn't it? I suspect this was the bank's master plan all along.

The second time was a result of being distracted by a child who had fallen and started wailing.

Needless to say, on both occasions, by the time I remembered and sprinted back, my money, which had grown tired of waiting for me, had decided to leave with someone else.

THE RIGHT SHI(F)**T:**
Blame the process, not the person

Never withdraw $80 from a cash machine. OK, maybe this time it was actually my fault and not the dollar amount.

Extending this idea to weight-loss . . .

That FAE insight is one of the most brilliant concepts I have ever come across and the possible applications are limitless.

While I didn't make this connection until many months after I read the book, I had this thought one day . . .

> *"If I make errors in attributing people's behavior to the way they are rather than the situation they are in, then it would be logical to assume I do the same thing with myself."*

That was really a critical insight for me and my weight-loss journey because I knew that FAE was definitely a factor in my lack of success over the past twenty-five years.

A simpler way to look at this . . .

I took the Heaths' FAE insight, turned the spotlight directly on myself, and asked this question:

> *Was it not possible that a problem I thought was a "ME" problem could in fact be a situation or a system problem?*

In looking back at my lack of success, it now seemed clear that I was making some grossly inaccurate assumptions.

Identifying "me" problems . . .

So I started looking at places where previous "me" problems might be system or situational problems and what I could implement to correct them.

Here were three I found, as well as the tweaks I made.

Me problem #1 . . .

No self-control when it came to eating junk food that was in my home.

I have no off switch when it comes to consuming junk food that finds its way into my house. I eat everything immediately (minus the packaging). For bulk items that I couldn't finish in one go, like a box of cereal, I would wake up in the middle of the night to polish off a few more bowls so that in the morning I would then be able to successfully finish off the remainder. That's insane, isn't it?

After giving this some thought, I realized this was *not* a "me" problem, but rather a system problem.

System Fix: *Junk the junk food.*

While this was a tough decision to make, I decided to eliminate the problem by completely banning junk food from the house. If I were going to have a treat, I would now have to travel to a destination in order to get it.

That solution has done wonders for me and made me realize self-control is really about developing strategies that allowed me to resist temptation. By removing the problem I no longer had a problem.

Me problem #2 . . .

I don't have the discipline to commit to an eating plan
or an eating schedule.

For as long as I can remember, I have wanted to create a weekly eating plan for myself and track the foods I ate so I could see what worked for me and what didn't. I would always start the process but never finish it.

The real problem was that logging my foods everyday was a big pain in the ass when I was simply using a spreadsheet. It was time-consuming and, worse, it wasn't really giving me any kind of feedback that could help me eat better.

I again realized I had falsely assumed I wasn't disciplined. But what if the solution I had defaulted to simply didn't work for what I was trying to do?

System Fix: *Find a software solution that made it easy and*
gave me usable feedback.

You have to love the times we live in now. While technology certainly comes with its challenges, it also comes with some massive upside if used properly.

I decided that I needed to find something that made the recording of foods easier, but more importantly, brought the information to life by giving me specific feedback I could monitor (more on this in another shift when I talk about carb control).

I eventually found a free online tool that not only allowed me to record my foods each day, but it also gave me a breakdown of the macronutrients I was consuming.

Me Problem #3 . . .

I graze to the point of overeating.

When I am at home, my inner cow takes over and I find myself constantly grazing on healthy foods. But too much of a healthy food is still too much food.

In this case, my food of choice was raw almonds. I keep them in my kitchen on a shelf in a see-through jar. Whenever I enter the kitchen, I can see them and instinctively reach in and grab a handful.

Those handfuls add up, and I find that a week's worth of nuts is gone in two or three days.

I now had enough experience to know I had a system problem.

System Fix: *Out of sight, out of mind.*

What I really had were two problems.

First, I can't eat foods in their bulk form. I need foods to be portioned beforehand, otherwise I will eat continuously until there is nothing left.

So my first decision was to divide my almonds up into 12 to 14 portions that were roughly a third of a cup. I then put them into tiny Tupperware containers, which have lids that are not transparent.

Second, I needed to remove the almonds from my field of vision. If I could see them, I would be drawn to them.

So I placed them into a much larger Tupperware container and then placed that on the back of the bottom shelf of my fridge.

And you know what? The problem was solved. For the first time ever, my week supply of almonds actually lasted eight days.

MAKE SHI(F)T HAPPEN...

1 Be open to the possibility (just plant the seed) that your "me" problems might actually be system problems. You will discover that more often than not, what you thought was a "me" problem is in fact a system problem. And your self-esteem will love you for that.

So when you have identified a problem, ask this question . . .

IS THIS A ME PROBLEM OR A SYSTEM PROBLEM?

---

2 When you discover a system problem, can it be solved by finding a way to hide it?

Simply putting something out of plain sight can go a long way. Burying something deep in the freezer, putting something in an out-of-reach cupboard, or storing stuff in a refrigerator that sits in your basement or garage may be all it takes to beat a problem that has plagued you for years.

MAKE THE VISIBLE INVISIBLE!

---

3 Can doing a little math solve a system problem? I added a software program to my life to take care of my discipline issue, and I removed junk food from the house to eliminate my self-control issue.

WHAT COULD YOU ADD OR SUBTRACT TO SOLVE YOUR PROBLEM?

Shift #3

DECIDE IN
ADVANCE ⇨

Without question, the worst experiences in my life are those that catch me completely off guard. I have run out of fingers and toes to keep track of all the stupid things I have either said (or forgotten to say) or done (or didn't do) because I was not prepared ahead of time to deal with potentially challenging situations.

For instance, I have gotten parking tickets because it never occurred to me to check and see if I had change with me before I left the house. I was then forced to play parking ticket roulette with the street-parking brigade. I lost more of those battles than I care to admit.

I have also been stranded in parking lots for hours because I locked my keys in my car (I once did this on consecutive days . . . DOH!). Having an extra key at home did little to help with those specific situations. It never occurred to me until much later to actually carry an extra key in my wallet, as the odds would be drastically reduced that I would lock both my keys and my wallet in the car together. (However, I once locked the keys in my car while it was running! Oh, and my wallet was resting comfortably on the passenger seat . . . double DOH!)

In both those cases, trouble could have easily been averted had I simply been proactive rather than reactive with my thinking. The mere act of thinking through what could go wrong in either of those situations and **deciding in advance** how I would behave would easily have eliminated the worst-case scenario.

Understandably, you can't anticipate everything that can happen in a particular situation. However, the more deliberate you are in thinking through potential pitfalls, the more success you will experience if and when things don't go according to plan.

MINDSHIFT: *Practice saves lives*

Amanda Ripley concludes *The Unthinkable: Who Survives When Disaster Strikes—and Why* by telling the story of Rick Rescorla.

You have probably never heard of Rescorla, but 2,687 survivors from 9/11 are alive because of his efforts.

Rescorla, a former Vietnam vet, was head of security for Morgan Stanley Dean Witter in Tower Two. After the 1993 truck bombing on the World Trade Center, Rescorla figured it was just a matter of time before terrorists would strike again. In fact, he wrote a report for Dean Witter executives outlining his fear of another attack. He even suggested that the towers were susceptible to an attack by plane.

Convinced, executives gave him more authority. He immediately started running regular fire drills with all members of the staff to ensure they knew what they should do in case of an emergency.

When he ran drills he would have the staff meet him in the hallway and at his direction enter the stairwell two by two. He timed them and trained them to exit faster. All the while, he used a bullhorn to bark instructions and keep people focused on what they were supposed to do.

The moment the first plane hit Tower One on the morning of September 11, 2001, Rescorla was ready and immediately sprang into action. With bullhorn in hand, he began marching his people down the stairwell like he had done for the previous eight years. Only this time it was no drill.

By the time Tower Two collapsed, all but thirteen who were employed by Dean Witter got out safely. Rescorla and four of his staff were among those who never made it out.

THE RIGHT SHI(F)T:
Have an action plan for eventualities

While this is an extreme example, Rescorla saved thousands by training people in advance on how to respond if an emergency should strike. Have action plans for the eventualities in your own life.

Going in blind...

I can honestly say that in my previous twenty-five years I had not once decided in advance how I might deal with potentially dicey situations, especially when it came to food that was destroying my body and my self-esteem.

I would simply show up at events and react to whatever stimulus was put in my face. The problem with this, however, was that my natural default tendencies sucked!

Consequently, any situations that I did not directly control usually resulted in a myriad of horrible decisions.

Did I want some pie? Hell yeah!

Did I want ice cream with that? Ah, hello! Pile on that Chunky Monkey, girlfriend.

Did I want the insanely large, impossible-to-finish popcorn for a mere $0.99 more? Abso-freaking-lutely!

As much joy as those offered for the ten or fifteen minutes they might last, the anguish and guilt I would later feel and have to live with for the remaining twenty-three hours and forty-five minutes of my day didn't seem to make these choices worthwhile.

And yet this pattern continued every time someone else controlled the menu.

I'm not the sharpest knife in the drawer, but even I knew I needed to put a new behavior in place if I was going to have any hope of creating sustainable, long-lasting change.

Deciding in advance...

In March of 2011, I was invited to a friend's fortieth birthday party. The party was being held at a local restaurant and was being catered, which meant there would be all kinds of wonderfully tantalizing foods available; most of which were no longer part of my food repertoire.

While I will talk about this in more detail in Shift #1: Go Paleo, I had given up foods that I had discovered were making me fat. So things like bread, pasta, and cakes (foods that I loved) were no longer part of my diet.

Though I was very much looking forward to the party, I was also worried about the relentless temptation that I would be faced with while I was there. History was not on my side.

So I decided to take an extraordinary measure. I would decide in advance how I was going to handle the various situations I inevitably knew would cross my path.

First, because the party was at 9 PM, I opted to eat my dinner as close to my departure time as possible so that I would not arrive hungry. I had done that way too many times in the past, and when I arrived I would eat like a bear getting ready for hibernation.

Second, since I knew I would be tempted by all the tasty treats, I brought a few small packs of raw almonds to have on hand when my friend, the munchies, showed up.

Third, I actually sat down and visualized how the night would unfold and how I would behave in a few precarious situations.

Up first was alcohol. It was a birthday party, so there would be lots. But alcohol and I have a rocky relationship. I don't like the chicken dance Alcohol-Me does, regardless of the musical genre. *Get with the times, Alcohol-Me. That is so 1980s.*

I like to shake hands with the new people I meet. Alcohol-Me likes to bear hug them and then pick them up off their feet and spin them around like they are Julie Andrews in *The Sound of Music* (so not cool).

I work hard to avoid junk food. Alcohol-Me, on the other hand, never tires of doing his impression of a bear at the dump eating all the garbage he can get his paws on.

So I decided I would only have one beer and drink water the rest of the night. Alcohol-Me wouldn't be happy, but I would make far better decisions as a result.

Next were all the tasty foods that were going to be served. I imagined myself simply saying "No, thank you." And this is exactly what I did.

'Would you like some little piggies in a blanket? No, thank you, my friend."

"How about these mini-hamburgers? No, thank you, good sir."

"Breaded cheese sticks? No, thank you, amigo."

That is how the whole night played out. I did not have a single finger food that was served. I snacked on a few nuts and some raw veggies.

The most unexpected event of the whole night was when I was leaving. My coat was right beside the birthday cupcakes they had for everyone. There I was, standing in front of these bad boys. And you know what? I didn't even have the urge to have one.

It was one of the most satisfying feelings I have ever had.

The night was a complete success, and looking back I realize it was all because I opted to **Decide in Advance** with regard to how I would respond to the eventualities.

MAKE SHI(F)T HAPPEN...

1 Watch this incredible talk by Sasha Dichter on TED. He was the inspiration behind the idea of deciding in advance. Have your pen and paper ready so you can borrow a few tips on how he used the strategy to enable him to become a more generous person.

The Generosity Experiment: www.ted.com/talks/sasha_dichter.html

DECIDING IN ADVANCE IS AN IDEA THAT TRANSCENDS BOUNDARIES!

---

2 Adopt a strategy from elite athletes: *Visualization!* They use it to ensure their success. Why would it be any different for you?

Book Recommendation: *Creative Visualization* by Shakti Gawain.

USE THE POWER OF YOUR IMAGINATION TO CREATE THE OUTCOME THAT YOU WANT!

3 Create a list of other areas where deciding in advance can help you achieve what you want. Here are other areas where I apply it:

✓ Going to a restaurant (I use the restaurant's online menu to determine what I will eat before I arrive)

✓ Going to someone's place for dinner (I send an email and tell them how I eat and ask what is on the menu)

✓ Traveling via airplane

✓ Driving a distance that takes longer than 60 minutes

✓ Being somewhere other than home for lunch or dinner

✓ Going to the movies

✓ Meeting friends for dinner and/or drinks

✓ Buying groceries

✓ Recovering from a bad eating day

✓ Creating my eating plan for the day/week

IDENTIFY AREAS IN YOUR LIFE WHERE YOU CAN APPLY "DECIDING IN ADVANCE!"

DISCOVER YOUR CARB THRESHOLD

When I decided in November 2010 that I once again wanted to try to change how I looked, I didn't have a clearly defined plan in place. Honestly, I had zero confidence that things would be any different from any other time I tried to lose weight. The big difference was I had already decided that if I was going to do another big face plant, I was going to do so implementing my own philosophy and my own ideas.

I mentioned in previous shifts that one of the first changes I embraced was the daily recording of all the foods I was eating. I didn't even change anything with my diet at that point.

I continued with my vegetarian ways, knowing that the simple act of recording everything I ate would instinctively lead me to make better, more informed food choices. This is one of the hidden benefits of recording. You gain the gift of mindfulness.

At the same time, I also started playing around with my workout philosophy, and after about a month I had begun to notice some small changes. They weren't massive by any stretch, but they were definitely noticeable to me.

I then had an unfortunate three-week period where I actually began to put weight back on. My initial thought at the time was, "Oh crap! Here we go again."

I must admit I was crushed by the setback, but after about thirty minutes of an f-bomb-filled internal shouting match, I realized that for the first time ever I had caught a problem in its infancy. This had never happened before.

Re-energized, I went back and looked at my food logs to see if I could find out what the hell went wrong. It didn't take long for me to find a scapegoat.

Damn you, Tim Ferriss . . .

In mid-December I started reading Tim Ferriss' new book, *The Four-Hour Body*. One of the things he discussed, which I wanted to test, was something he called the slow-carb breakfast.

My breakfast had been the same for the last five years. I always had a "healthy" fruit-based smoothie with some sort of protein additive.

Ferriss talked about a breakfast that was comprised of eggs, beans, and an assortment of veggies. Since I was still vegetarian, this fit perfectly into my eating philosophy, so I decided to give his breakfast a go.

But around the third week in January I noticed I was getting rather portly again (OK, OK! I was getting fat), and the only real change in my diet was the slow-carb breakfast. So I decided to abandon it completely and go back to my shakes for the remainder of the week.

But I was still intrigued by the idea of a slow-carb meal, so I started looking for resources on carbs to get a better understanding of how they impacted my body.

The results of my research were quite encouraging. The more I learned about carbs and their impact on the body, the more I realized that maybe, just maybe, this was where my problem lay.

A theory is born . . .

There are some people out there who strongly believe that the over-consumption of carbs is the cause of obesity. Logically, their solution suggests that if people want to stop being fat they should be eating a low-carb diet.

I had also seen a rash of foods on the market that were hyped as low-carb but were also high in crapola, so I was not sold on the notion that simply going low-carb was the way to go. For crying out loud, Diet Coke is low-carb, but it still doesn't change the fact that it is liquid crap in a can.

I also knew that every single diet approach I had seen made the same fundamental error. It assumed everyone's body responded the exact same way to a particular stimulus. This is just silly, of course. A diet (a way of eating) has to be catered specifically to the person and not to an entire population.

So I formulated a different theory by asking a different question.

What if each person has a carb threshold?

For some that threshold might be incredibly high, meaning they have a very forgiving body type when it comes to eating a diet high in carbs. Consequently, these people can get away with eating things like breads, pastas, etc. without the threat of weight gain, disease, or illness.

For others (the majority it seems), that threshold is considerably lower because their body type is particularly carb-sensitive. So these people have significantly less wiggle room in the carb department and, as a result, gain weight easily when that threshold is breached.

This made perfect sense in my case. My vegetarian diet was super-high in carbs. On an average day I was consuming 300–450grams of carbs, which is very high. Not only did I suspect I was breaching my carb threshold, I was stampeding right through it.

This was a critical insight for me, which allowed me to begin asking a set of more specific questions directed toward me. The most important of which was this:

Was it possible I was flooding my body with way too many carbs, thus preventing it from shedding the body fat it so desperately wanted to shed?

A different kind of apple...

With the idea of a carb threshold in mind, I continued to do more research, looking for something that might help me make all this more tangible and actionable.

Somehow I ended up on Mark Sisson's blog, *Mark's Daily Apple*, where I found a post with the following chart.

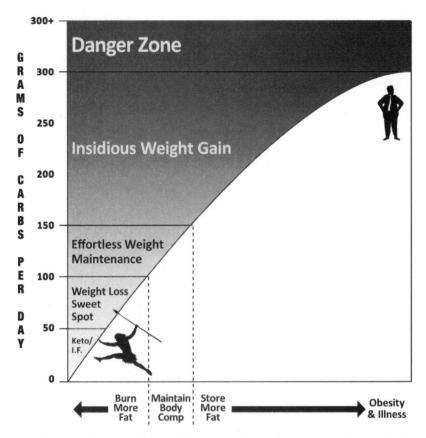

(©Mark Sisson as found in The Primal Blueprint (2009), used by permission. Thanks Mark!)

It gave me the very thing I was looking for. I now had something tangible that I could test.

Make no mistake. I was not blindly accepting this chart as gospel. I was no longer assuming anything. If an idea made sense to me in theory, then and only then would I test it on myself to see if it had any merit.

As you can see from the chart, it suggests that keeping your daily carb total somewhere between 50g and 100g is optimal for fat loss. Weight can be maintained if you hover between 100g and 150g of carbs. The tendency to store fat increases the further one climbs above the 150g mark.

Yikes! If the theory was correct, I had some idea of why I was fat. In fact, with the amount of carbs I was consuming each day I was surprised I was not the size of a hot air balloon.

Where to begin?

I must admit the chart fascinated me. But as I stated above, I was also wary. Just because someone says it is so, doesn't make it so. Too many of us make that mistake. Experts are people and they too have agendas and biases and can slant information to prove something they believe in strongly.

Keeping this in mind, I needed to test this idea for myself to see if it made sense for my body type. The theory certainly seemed plausible based on my particular set of circumstances.

My bigger problem, though, resulted from the fact that I had no idea what the chart meant in terms of how a typical eating day might look for me. What the hell could I eat that would come within the accepted carb range?

And so I began to test, but with the following rules in place:

First, I was not going to starve myself. I didn't want to look like one of those hyenas you see on the Discovery Channel who are all emaciated and always hovering around food. I don't need to run a study to know that starvation diets are *not* sustainable.

Second, I was going to eat six times per day. This meant I would eat every three hours, and ensure I wouldn't go hungry. In fact, one of my new commandments was, **NEVER BE HUNGRY!**

BULLSHI(F)T: *When the "experts" stack the deck against your success*

I had an e-mail exchange with a girl I used to go to university with. I had not talked with her in about twenty-five years and it brought back a flood of great memories. She was a wonderful girl, and pretty too.

But she suffered the same fate I suffered back then. Our unforgiving bodies started storing more body fat than we would have liked while we were in our early twenties.

She mentioned that this was something she had continued to battle twenty-five years later. When I inquired how that battle was going, she mentioned that she was working with a professional in the industry and this is what the "expert" had convinced her to accept:

"It's OK for me to go to bed hungry."

I remember reading that and feeling both sad and frustrated. That's the stupidest advice you could ever give someone. It's *not* OK to go to bed hungry. First, if you are hungry, then there is a hole in your diet. Somehow what you are eating is not nourishing your body, causing you to feel unsatisfied.

Second, going to bed hungry is *not* sustainable long-term. The energy required to fight your natural urges every single night is impossible to sustain, for the mere fact that you have limited energy reserves to begin with. This is why your body is telling you it's hungry in the first place.

Sadly, there are a lot of "experts" out there who are dishing out advice they themselves don't follow. As I have stated in previous shifts, much of this has to do with the fact that a great many don't understand their own success.

> **THE RIGHT SHI**(F)**T:** *Sustainability is the name of the game*
>
> When adopting new behaviors, you need to think in terms of sustainability by asking this question: "Can I still be doing this five years from now?" If the answer is no, it isn't sustainable. If it isn't sustainable, *Don't do it*!

Big changes on the horizon . . .

I set about researching foods and their carb content to see what I could throw together that would allow me to meet all of my eating criteria while coming within an acceptable, albeit arbitrary, carb range for my body.

As I began to research individual foods and food combinations, I was amazed at some of the things I discovered. Here are a few:

Thing #1: Fruit was killing me! Single servings of fruits like bananas (I ate at least two a day) and apples were really high in carbs. Two bananas and an apple would put me at 100 grams of carbs for the day. Whoa!

Thing #2: Bread products (which I loved) were really high in carbs. I had known for a long time that bread always left me feeling fat and bloated, so this was not a big shocker.

Thing #3: Beans and legumes were also super-high in carbs. This now made sense, considering I had just discovered that beans made me fat. Who knew?

Thing #4: Good protein sources (organic, free-range, grass-fed) like chicken, lean meats, and fish had almost zero carbs. This was nice to know.

Thing #5: Not all carbs are created equal (good carbs vs. bad carbs). Just because something is low in carbs doesn't mean it is something I should be eating. This would be a particularly important distinction when it came to evaluating processed foods.

Thing #6: It's not about a diet low in fat; it's about a diet that has a healthy dose of good fats. This was a big shift for sure because I, like everyone else out there, was under the illusion that fat makes you fat. *FYI: It does not.*

So with my newfound knowledge in hand, I set about making some drastic changes to my diet.

First, I decided that I would keep my carb count around 100grams of carbs each day. Since these numbers were rather arbitrary, I thought I would start with that and then see what worked for my body type.

Second, if I wanted to accomplish the first, I couldn't do it eating a plant-based diet. So I pulled the plug on being vegetarian. It was clear that it just wasn't working for my body type. And so, after almost nineteen years, I decided that I would reintroduce quality meats to my diet.

Jump ahead about two months and the unthinkable happened. For the very first time in my life, I actually saw my abs.

MAKE SHI(F)T HAPPEN...

1 Make the decision to start logging what you eat each and every day. Great companies don't happen by accident. Neither do great bodies. The mere act of being mindful of what you are eating will have a massive impact on your health.

TRACK WHAT YOU EAT DAILY!

2 For the next week or two, don't change anything in your diet. Simply record everything you are eating and drinking. The reason for this is you want comparison data. Then you can start making tweaks slowly and methodically.

DON'T MAKE ANY CHANGES UNTIL YOU HAVE A CLEAR SENSE OF WHERE YOU ARE!

3 When you are ready to start, see where your average carb threshold used to be and see if that needs to be tweaked. You can use the chart as a guide, or use your own ideas. But start somewhere and test relentlessly. As you progress, the goal is to find out where your threshold lies.

DISCOVER YOUR CARB THRESHOLD!

Shift #1

GO PALEO ➡

Before you read more about the numero uno shift I made to finally get the body I long desired, I want to make this very clear. I do not believe that there is one universal diet (a way of eating) that will work for everyone. To make such a claim would assume that everyone reacts exactly the same to every stimulus they encounter.

That's just crazy talk. That would be like saying everyone exposed to the flu virus will get the flu (only a small percentage do), or that everyone who watches a comedy will all laugh at the same scenes (they don't), or that everyone who reads this book is going to agree with everything I say. I'm kidding on this last one. Of course everyone will agree with everything I say. I wrote a book about it. I can't be wrong, right?

My point is to make you aware that we are extremely complex individuals. One "diet" *cannot* possibly satisfy all our needs. (It is important for me to note here that I do not consider paleo a diet, but rather a lifestyle and a way of living.)

This one-size-fits-all mentality that people and corporations use to sell product is strategically flawed thinking because it ignores our complexity. Yet that is exactly the kind of thinking that exists on either side of the weight-loss (read as body transformation) equation.

People with weight-loss products prey on those desperate for change by promoting universal solutions (meaning they imply what they offer will help anyone who is struggling). On the other side, people struggling with getting the body they want assume there is only ONE answer out there and simply jump from one universal cure to the next, hoping that next cure is THE THING that will finally help them solve their problem.

But that kind of thinking is terribly flawed and incredibly destructive. There are far better ways to build a lifestyle approach to body transformation, but in order to do this, you need to understand how we acquire knowledge.

MINDSHIFT: *Read the small print*

Ever watch the TV commercials of companies that offer weight-loss solutions? You know the ones I am talking about.

Even they know that their product only works for a select group of people. They know that even if a person follows the program as prescribed, there is a good chance they won't experience the advertised results.

How do we know they know? Because after they promote the very best examples they have (or skip real testimonials in favor of paid actors), there is a little disclaimer in itsy bitsy writing that says . . .

THESE RESULTS ARE NOT TYPICAL!

Of course they don't run that little bit of information until after they've hooked you with their cleverly crafted pitch. By that time, they know most people who are desperate for change won't even see the small print (or hear the warning) or will simply ignore it.

My bigger question is, "If the results are not typical, why are you showing them in the first place?" The answer? To mislead you, of course.

Weight-loss companies are not the only ones who attempt to deceive people with clever marketing ploys to draw attention away from the fact that the product they offer is average at best.

A very popular golfer (whom I quite like) endorses an arthritis product for a condition he suffers from. The thing runs like an SNL skit. I actually went to the company website and wrote down the side effects that are read during the commercial while the golfer is shown playing outside with his children and enjoying his life.

These are the side effects as read by the narrator . . .

. . . it may lower your ability to fight infections; serious, sometimes FATAL events including infection, tuberculosis, lymphoma, other cancers and nervous system and blood disorders have occurred. Tell your doctor . . .

[Capitals and bold on the word fatal were mine.]

So the last time I checked, I am pretty sure FATAL means you WILL die. So if I understand correctly, this company is putting out a drug that might lessen your arthritis pain, but there is a chance it will kill you as well.

I'm not a doctor, but I'm pretty sure death lessens arthritic pain as well, so I guess one way or the other they are correct.

> **THE RIGHT SHI**(F)**T:** *Be an educated consumer*
>
> The next time you are watching TV, keep an eye out for the commercials that promote a cure to a chronic issue. As you view it, watch how they communicate their message that "results are not typical."

A paradigm shift is needed!

If I could get you to walk away with just one idea it would be this: A healthy lifestyle is put together like the knowledge you possess.

It comes from everything you have ever been exposed to. Your cumulative knowledge base is *not* the university or college you went to (I pride myself on the fact the only thing I learned in university was how to drink beer through a garden hose). In fact, your formal education plays a negligible role in the overall acquisition of knowledge and insight you possess.

You have acquired far more from:

⇨ Your parents

⇨ Your peers, work colleagues, and mentors you interact with

⇨ The work that you do

⇨ The books, magazines, and blogs you read

⇨ The movies and shows you watch

⇨ The performances and seminars you attend

⇨ The websites you visit (i.e. www.TED.com)

⇨ The personal insights you discover

⇨ The experiences you have

⇨ The places you travel

That is exactly how great health is assembled. It is woven together from an incredibly diverse selection of exceptionally reliable sources.

Of all the things on that list, the experiences I've had were by far the most significant in shaping the program I created for myself. So let me walk you through the chronology of my dietary evolution.

A diet of all seasons...

One of the unique perspectives I bring to all this is that I have lived five very distinct diets over the course of my lifetime.

Notice I used the verb "lived" and not "eaten." Living a diet allows me to discuss things from a unique perspective. I am not claiming that makes me an expert, but I have credibility and can draw on my own vast experiences to help others solve their problems.

Season #1

For the first twenty-two years of my life I ate a conventional diet, which consisted of *a lot of* processed foods. It also included essential staples like Fruit Loops, Kraft Mac & Cheese, and the god of late-night snacks, the grilled cheese sandwich.

Result: 50 to 60 pounds overweight as I crept up to 215 pounds of nasty goo.

Season #2 (about three years)

When that didn't work, I decided to pull red meat from my diet, opting to eat only chicken and fish on occasion.

And you will never guess why I took red meat out of my diet? Because I heard a study on the radio that said red meat was bad for you. I was such an idiot back then (I am less so now). *No one* should blindly accept a study until they have analyzed it themselves based on their own criteria of what constitutes good science. Sadly, I had no such parameters at that time.

Result: 30 to 40 pounds overweight, depending on whether gravity was out to get me or not.

Season #3 (about five years on and off)

I then transitioned from that into full-fledged veganism. This meant *no* animal products at all. Actually, in the true sense of the word, vegans are also not supposed to wear animal products.

Result: 20 to 40 pounds overweight, depending on the month.

Season #4 (about fifteen years)

I then loosened the reins on my militant vegan stance and added things like eggs and dairy back into my diet. I was a real vegetarian (as opposed to the pretend, fair-weather vegetarians that occasionally eat meat like chicken and fish).

Result: 20 to 40 pounds overweight, no matter how much exercise I did.

Season #5 (Present)

On January 27, 2011, I decided to ditch the vegetarian diet. Fifteen years was more than enough time for me to realize that vegetarianism did not work for my body type.

I quickly transitioned into eating a paleo-like diet (aka the caveman diet). I introduced some quality meats back in and took all grains, sugars, food additives, and crappy fats out.

Result: weight-loss of 40 to 45 pounds
(This is an approximation because I don't weigh myself, but after about two months of eating super-clean I could actually see my abs.)

Vegetarianism, you're fired!

So why did I axe vegetarianism? Because I finally decided to evaluate it based on my own personal experience, and the truth was that the diet never did work for me. It didn't matter what the science and the literature stated. The truth was I gave it a serious go and it didn't work for my body type.

I am well aware that this statement leaves me vulnerable to those who are passionate about this way of eating. Some will attempt to wade in and diagnose my "real" problem without knowing anything about me or how I lived.

Those individuals will suggest I was eating too much. Others will probably allude to the notion that I must have been eating a lot of junk food or other processed foods, and the fitness fanatics will conclude that I was not engaging in enough exercise.

Let me address each of these arguments.

First, with regard to overeating, it could have been possible that I was eating too much. However, I eat more now than I did then, so that line of logic is squashed.

With regard to processed foods, my philosophy remains the same as it was then. The bulk of my vegetarian diet was raw, mostly organic whole foods from natural sources. The only processed food I occasionally ate was organic salsa, tuna packed in water, and a variety of vegetarian "meat" products (that I had long suspected were making me fat).

My junk food was limited as well. Each week I would have ice cream, along with some organic corn chips and salsa.

And with regards to exercise, well, I have always been active. I would do something three to five times a week and it was always pretty intense. So that argument didn't hold much water, either. In fact, I work out less now then I did before, so again, the logic is flawed.

Why labels are bad...

If I am no longer vegetarian, what the hell am I?

I'm reluctant to put a label on how I eat now because the moment you label something, you invariably invite debate, and I have no intention of defending my dietary choices to anyone.

I couldn't care less what others think of my eating lifestyle, nor do I feel the need to convince them I am right. I only need to convince myself what is right and what isn't in my pursuit of optimal health. It is a challenge at times to stay true to this. As humans, there is an innate desire to try and please others. I have had to work hard to not give a rat's ass what others think in this domain.

But for all my talk about not liking labels, the way I eat and the lifestyle I engage in does have a name. Some knuckle draggers refer to it as the caveman diet. It is more commonly referred to as the paleo diet, in reference to the period of time the diet was most prevalent: the Paleolithic era.

Paleo 101...

To simplify things here, I will stick with the phrase paleo diet. Wikipedia does a great job capturing the essence of it.

> *The Paleolithic diet, also popularly referred to as the caveman diet, Stone Age diet, and hunter-gatherer diet, is a nutritional plan based on the presumed ancient diet of wild plants and animals that various human species habitually consumed during the Paleolithic era—a period of about 2.5 million years duration that ended around 10,000 years ago with the development of agriculture. The diet consists mainly of grass-fed pasture-raised meats, fish, vegetables, fruit, roots, and nuts, and excludes grains, legumes, dairy products, salt, refined sugar, and processed oils.*

I don't want to turn this into a history lesson (mainly because my ability to correctly recite historical facts is as good as my ability to get the words to a song correct . . . it doesn't happen often), but roughly 10,000 years ago we saw the first signs of agriculture appear.

This was the beginning of humans moving away from the hunting and gathering mentality and moving toward the domestication of plants and animals and husbands (the jury is still out on the last one).

Just so we are all on the same page, allow me to highlight the obvious. We ate a Paleolithic diet for roughly 2,500,000 years. In the last 10,000 years we have introduced grains, processed foods, and food additives, among other things.

Our genes were programmed to function a certain way for 2.5 million years. The last 10,000 years we have been trying to rewrite the code by asking them to function in a new way. This new approach to eating represents only 0.4% of our timeline as eaters.

Now the pro-paleo tribe contends that there are people who suffer sensitivities to these new foods due to their relative newness on our evolutionary timeline. There is a line of thinking (and studies as well) that suggests the rise in obesity, disease, and illness correlates with this advent of agriculture.

The paleo approach recommends that these people (suffering from any or all of the above) would do much better on a diet that accommodates our evolutionary ancestry and suggests eliminating grains, legumes, dairy products, salt, refined sugar, and processed oils from one's diet.

Making up my own mind...

I stated in Shift #19 that I ignore most experts. But what do I do with those experts I don't ignore? Well, for those I have to filter their message through my own philosophy to see what makes sense and what doesn't. And that is precisely what I did when I stumbled upon the paleo diet.

For instance, I was under no illusions that much of the information about man (and his smarter half, woman) for the past 2.5 million years is observational in nature. No one knows for certain exactly how they lived back then, so any references to how they ate, how healthy they were, what the average lifespan was, and what diseases did or did not exist were purely hypothetical in nature (for the most part).

That said, it made sense to me on an intellectual level that the Fred Flintstones of our past ate a diet based on what they had access to, and, having done so for 2.5 million years, it seemed logical that optimal gene expression could be enhanced by a diet that was more in line with our evolutionary ancestry.

Seriously, there are all kinds of other aspects of my life that have an evolutionary mechanism at play. For instance, I duck, jump, or scream (in a manly fashion, of course) when I am startled. Why couldn't my diet also reflect this mechanism?

Another paleo-centric argument revolved around the elimination of certain foods. Because the by-products of agriculture are relatively new on our evolutionary scale, the question that arises is, "Should everyone then eliminate grains, legumes, dairy products, salt, refined sugar, and processed oils from their diet?" Again, I filtered this through my own philosophy.

Personally, I believe refined sugars along with processed foods and their additives are literally killing people. I had removed most of that crap years ago. Those are things I would strongly recommend anyone remove, regardless of what diet they adopt.

Do I believe everyone must remove grains, legumes, and dairy from their diet? Of course not! Not everyone on the planet has issues with these foods. We are as different as our DNA.

Do I think more people should give this lifestyle a try? Based on what I am seeing from the general population on a day-to-day basis, abso-freaking-lutely. You don't need to possess a doctorate degree to realize we have an obesity epidemic on our hands. But people must make that call for themselves based on their unique biological differences.

I made a decision based on the symptoms I had experienced from my previous diets. There was ample evidence to suggest that dairy, legumes, and grains were altering my body type. So the paleo solution seemed like a logical hypothesis to test. The key word there is test. I was not blindly going to accept anything as fact. I would test and tweak and see what worked for my particular body type.

And the results...

Well, if you saw my shameless promotional pics at the beginning of the book, I think the results speak for themselves. The paleo diet has allowed my genes to express their true nature, and I have been able to transform myself into someone I had never before seen.

MAKE SHI(F)T HAPPEN...

1 Listen, I don't care what path you choose to travel, because at the end of the day I have no control over your choices. **BUT YOU DO!** Don't let someone else determine your fate. Decide for yourself. Be the pilot of your own plane, the captain of your own ship, the handler of your own luggage. *Think about that last one. You never have to deal with lost baggage when you only have carry-on.*

TEST YOUR OWN HYPOTHESIS & COMMIT TO MAKING UP YOUR OWN MIND!

2 If you are at the point where you have exhausted your resources and are desperate to try something else that actually makes sense and is sustainable long-term, I suggest you learn as much as you can about the paleo diet. *But* act now.

It's easy to get caught up researching, but researching is not action. Start now. Start doing something. Anything. Remove sugar from your coffee. Stop drinking pop (soda for those who don't live in Canada). Make your own salad dressing, as opposed to using one loaded with garbage.

Here are the three sites I highly recommend to get you started. Each has a book as well.

Sarah Fragoso of www.everydaypaelo.com; Book: *Everyday Paleo* (National bestseller)

Robb Wolf of www.robbwolf.com; Book: *The Paleo Solution* (*NY Times* bestseller)

Mark Sisson of www.marksdailyapple.com; Book: *The Primal Blueprint*

EDUCATE YOURSELF, BUT START TAKING MEASURABLE ACTION NOW!

---

3 If you opt to commit to giving paleo a try, then understand there is no in-between with this. You can't be a little bit pregnant, and you can't be a little bit paleo (but you can be a little rock and roll). You are either all-in or all-out.

Speaking from my own experience, I went all-in right away. I excluded grains, legumes, dairy products, salt, refined sugar, and processed oils. And you know what? It took about two months to see results, but it worked!

DIETS ARE LIKE ONE NIGHT STANDS. GOING PALEO IS LIKE GETTING MARRIED. YOU'RE IN IT FOR THE LONG HAUL.

When SHI(F)T happens

FROM WOE TO WOW!

Going from 195 pounds to 141 pounds ⇨

Laurie Anne's Story...

Laurie Anne is a subscriber on my blog. She sent me a wonderful follow-up e-mail detailing her own experiences with the paleo lifestyle. What surprised me the most was that she didn't write to tell me her tale of woe. She wrote me to tell me her tale of WOW!

I loved it! This woman was e-mailing to tell me how she had **MADE SHI**(F)**T HAPPEN!**

There was something awesome about her writing style. She was funny and articulate, and it was clear she had a much deeper understanding of this process than most. So I probed a little deeper (but not in an alien abduction kind of way) to see what insights she had learned along the way.

In our second e-mail exchange, she took the liberty to send me a before-and-after picture. I was stunned! This woman had gone from 194 pounds to 141 pounds in about five months, and she had done so in a smart, sustainable fashion while overcoming some gigantic obstacles.

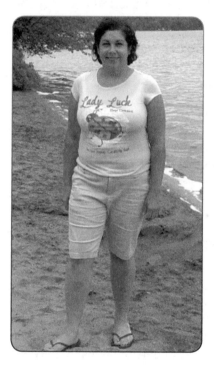 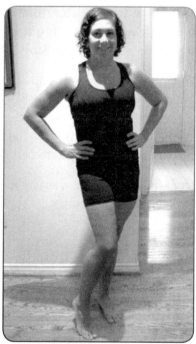

8 days, 10 questions...

I knew I needed to capture Laurie Anne's story, but I wanted to do it properly. As I have said previously, too many people aren't even aware of the factors responsible for their own success, so it's hard for them to describe the key points to their progress. Instead, most focus on tired clichés and catch phrases. These are not helpful to others looking for clues to help in their own quest to transform their bodies.

What people really need are details, and they need answers to real concerns. Why did you know this time would be different? Do you still struggle? How do you pick yourself up when you fail? What do you do when you have cravings? How do you deal with people who are not supportive?

It was clear from my e-mail exchanges with Laurie Anne that she knew how to tell a story that would do more than simply inspire people. It would shed insight and provide those valuable clues that others were seeking. Her story would change lives.

We agreed to do an in-depth e-mail interview where I would ask her ten questions. She could answer them any way she wanted (no censoring or filtering on my part), with as much detail as she felt was needed. I would then craft a follow-up question based on her previous response, adding a little commentary and insight of my own.

Our e-mail exchange went on for eight days. It exceeded my wildest expectations.

Learn from her story...

There are many shifts that Laurie Anne has used that parallel mine. But there are others that are uniquely hers. And that is awesome, because it reinforces the notion that each person needs to piece together their own unique plan to **MAKE SHI**(F)**T HAPPEN!**

So allow me to make a suggestion here.

Plan to read her story at least two times. The first time through, read it to simply be inspired by her success, knowing that change is possible for you as well. But understand that inspiration is perishable. You need more than inspiration to allow you to **MAKE SHI**(F)**T HAPPEN!**

The second time through, put the inspiration aside and become the student. Grab a pen or a highlighter and start underlining ideas worth appropriating. Take note of situations that parallel your story (this is important because we often feel very alone when we are attempting to make change).

I would also encourage you to seek out the specific shifts she used to help her create the transformation she created. And then borrow some as you attempt to create your own unique plan to **MAKE SHI**(F)**T HAPPEN!**

Laurie Anne's amazing transformation...

Subject: Question #1

Hey Laurie Anne,

Wowzers! Your transformation has been amazing.

So with question #1 I would like you to give us some context about your weight-loss struggles.

For instance, have you always struggled with your weight? When did it start becoming a problem? How were you dealing with it at that time? Feel free to take the question in any direction you want.

DD

Subject: Response to Question #1

Have I struggled with my weight? YES! I have battled with my weight all my life, but more so in the few years after my firstborn. I remember loving the excuse, "I just had a baby," which at some point didn't fly, like when my son was five years old.

I was always the girl with the pretty face, which we all know is "code" for "she'd be gorgeous if she wasn't so fat."

Two pregnancies later and much heavier, I became an avid baker. I loved to sample my treats before I served them, and on many occasions would inhale the whole creation, taking extra care to hide any evidence. . . . I felt like a thief and was ashamed . . . yet I did it again and again!

Five years ago I became a vegetarian in an effort to get healthy, lose some weight, and try to fight the constant bloat I was always experiencing, which, by the way, my doctor alleged was due to my high-fat, high-meat diet.

I was diagnosed with depression and high blood pressure and, highly medicated, I just kept getting heavier. As long as the sizes in the store could keep accommodating me, I felt like I was not alone in my struggles. There were others my size . . . how bad could it be?

By December of 2010, my weight was 185 pounds; I was still five-foot-five. I was on the treadmill six days a week and was put on a low-fat, low-carb diet by my doctor, who was dead against the vegetarian diet I had been on previously and blamed my medical issues on it.

"Fine! I'll try it his way" was my reaction, but in a mere ten months I had gained another ten pounds. WTF? How could that be? I felt like crap, I looked like crap, and if I complained to the doctor he just upped my meds, which in turn made me feel worse! And now on top of all that I was developing high cholesterol as well.

I had no confidence to speak of, never have in my adult life. I have always had a hard time accepting compliments of any sort. After all, how could anyone like me if I, in fact, hated myself.

I remember feeling paralyzed in social situations, ashamed and wanting to hide. I wanted to climb up into the bell tower of Notre Dame and kick Quasimodo out! Why did he hide? A measly hump on his back! I am the one who needed to hide.

Yeah . . . I know a little bit about struggling with weight.

Subject: Question #2

Hey Laurie Anne,

Well first, I will never look at Quasimodo the same again. What a whiner he was! Dude, it's a hump. You probably still have a six-pack in that twisted up body of yours!

And I can definitely relate to the "working your ass off" and having nothing to show for it.

If my timeline is right, that took you into late February/early March of 2011, and you are now 195 pounds (I'm showing off my third-grade math skills here).

So with my second question, clearly something pivotal (a powerful inciting incident) happened at this time. Spill the beans. What was it?

DD

Subject: Response to Question #2

Right you are Dean! 195 pounds! By mid-February 2011. Your third-grade math teacher would be so proud!

So by February I was feeling the lowest I had ever felt, and my doctor started talking about putting me on statins for my high cholesterol. I freaked out! I was already on anti-depressants, high blood pressure meds, a water pill. I ate Advil like it was candy for every little pain. And I seemed to have a lot of pain regularly—body aches, headaches . . . I was a mess!

My grandmother died in her sixties, my mother is in her sixties, and I was following in their footsteps both physically and medically. I visited my mother just before Valentine's Day to bring over some chocolates and took one look at her and it was as if I saw her in a different light. She had trouble getting out of her chair to greet us, she had no energy, and seemed to have just lost that lust for life. It was at that moment that I decided to do something about it.

I was not going to end up like them! I wanted to live, laugh, and love myself.

I am the type of person that always goes whole hog when I do something. I don't eat one cookie; I eat twelve. I don't ease into a diet; I throw myself into it. So discovering the primal diet through a friend who mentioned she was going to give it a whirl made me curious, and I Googled it, went to the bookstore and read about it, and inhaled as much info as I could about the primal/paleo lifestyle.

It was just the medicine I needed! Something so radically out there that it might just work!

I talked to my doctor about it, who immediately reacted negatively, just as I had assumed he would (which only made me want to do it even more!) I was tired of his solutions, which got me nowhere.

And so . . . I jumped in!

Subject: Question #3

Hey Laurie Anne,

First, I admire you HUGELY for ignoring your doctor. I'm not saying people should, but people forget not all doctors are created equal. I want a doctor who says, "Listen, we need to get you better so you are not on medication." Not someone who does the reverse.

That takes tremendous guts, Laurie. That's a huge lesson in taking ownership. You are first in the chain of command. People (including doctors) can make suggestions, but we decide what direction our health is going to go.

> So two things come to mind for question #3.
>
> 1. What did you read? Were there a few specific sources that you found influential?
>
> 2. Elaborate on "Jumped in!"
>
> DD

Subject: Response to Question #3

I ignored my doctor. In fact, as I was leaving his office I was already scheming never to return. Don't get me wrong, he's a great guy, just antiquated in his views and unwilling to consider that maybe, just maybe, there could be new evidence to suggest that some things he learned from his textbook in university have changed drastically.

My doctor himself is not the picture of perfect health.

I got home, made a cup of tea, and didn't put my usual Sweet'N Low substitute in it . . . prepared it black and sat at the counter with the laptop. I typed in "Paleo" or "Primal diet" and the first thing I clicked on was a link to *The Paleo Solution* by Robb Wolf . . . a great starting point for me.

I read the site thoroughly and found it all fascinating, but what I liked most was the forum. I liked to read other peoples experiences; it made it less scary and acted kind of like peer pressure for me. If they're all doing it, why can't I? I signed up for the forum and picked peoples' brains.

Somewhere in that frame of time I tried, really tried, to drink my tea, but it was disgusting! I dumped it out and headed to my local library.

The library had no books on the paleo or primal way of life, but what I did manage to find were some grain-free cookbooks, as well as the Atkins series. I figured that getting lists of low-carb foods was a great place to start for a newbie like myself.

It all exhausted me. I came home that day, drew a bath, and cried. . .

Could I do this? Was it safe? Why bother? After all nothing else had worked.

I talked to my hubby about it. He was very skeptical and borderline angry that I would want to do something so "dangerous." A "high-fat, high-protein diet would kill me," were his choice words of encouragement.

Call me crazy! But this just pushed me into it! I would show everyone!

In the forums I had read that some people plan a start date and ease into it slowly, others vow to do a thirty-day challenge. I jumped in. In my soul I think I started the moment my friend had told me to look into this diet because she'd heard great things about it. In my heart I started the moment I opted to not put the sweetener in my tea.

And so I started drinking green tea and only having one black tea a day with a touch of cream. No more bread—lettuce became my bread of choice. No more baked goods. I opted for blueberries and nuts for sweet treats. And I began to eat eggs and bacon and more vegetables than I had eaten as a vegetarian.

I cleaned the pantry and refrigerator and made space for my new groceries that I would need.

Within the first two weeks I lost an amazing 9 pounds . . . two weeks! What was fantastic was not the numbers, but the fact that my clothes were a little loose. Nothing could wipe the grin off my face. This made me stronger in my convictions. I was ready to fight this thing and win this time!

Armed with a notebook that contained lists of foods I could and couldn't eat, I went shopping and bought the foods that I would eat daily . . . blueberries, almonds, walnuts, spinach, peppers and other veggies, eggs, meat, chicken and fish, green tea, almond butter, olive oil, coconut oil, and a whole coconut. This was exciting!

Subject: Question #4

Hey Laurie Anne,

I said it before Laurie, but man oh man, you know how to tell a story. Seriously, this is like Harry Potter gone primal (or wild?) . . . the nonfiction version, mind you.

I'm also SO amazed by your ability to be undaunted by those around you who were all saying, "Don't do it." Isn't it interesting how so many people claim to be experts on diet, yet very few actually look the part. The problem is most of us make the *stupid* mistake of listening to them.

I also think there is a subtle brilliance to just jumping in. People find ways to put it off, or subconsciously talk themselves out of it, but it has been my experience that those who succeed, JUMP IN knowing this is a journey that *starts now* . . .

Here is something else you did that is brilliant . . . a LIST of foods you could and could NOT eat.

The more visual and real this is, the more likely this will happen. The list acts like street signage. People only stop when they see a stop sign (well, most people anyway). A list of foods not to eat creates the same response. Did I say that was brilliant! Oh, I did.

OK, so question #4 is for inquiring minds that want to know . . .

1. What was in your pantry that you tossed?

2. What is on your no-eat list?

3. Did this all happen on day one when you jumped in?

DD

Subject: Response to Question #4

My cooking repertoire as I knew it had to change; my taste buds had to undergo a transformation.

I emptied my pantry of flour, crackers, cookies, beans (oh, how I would miss chickpeas . . . or would I?) pasta, breadcrumbs, sugar, sugar substitutes, and any other packaged goodies I could find. I relegated my trusty bread maker (wouldn't be needing it again) and all my "treat" cookbooks to the basement (outta sight, outta mind).

But in all my excitement and determination I forgot one tiny detail. Well, maybe not so tiny . . . my family!

I already knew my husband wasn't on board. How would my fifteen-year-old and eleven-year-old cope with the changes? Was it safe for them? They are blessed with their father's speedy metabolism and slender physique.

The more I read about going grain-free, it wasn't just about weight-loss, but overall optimum health and an antidote for modern disease. So surely my family could only benefit . . . right?

It didn't go over well. The kids were very unsupportive and were downright livid when there was no rice/potato/pasta on their plate. And snacks were a nightmare! "What do you mean we can't have cookies or pizza pops?"

Normally this type of conflict would have me settle back into my old way of doing things . . . but there was something different about this.

I decided that they could continue eating whatever the h-e-double hockey sticks they wanted to. After all, this was the first time in my life that I was going to do something selfish, something just for me. In fact, in the space of one month while all this was transpiring, I had lost a total of 16 pounds. IT WAS WORKING! And this is all the push I needed to continue.

My clothes were loose. I began to measure my success by taking my measurements—chest, waist, hips . . . my clothes looked frumpy, but best of all I felt great! I was full of energy, almost manic. I had that joie de vivre I keep hearing so much about . . . and this was only the beginning. People began to notice and ask, "Have you lost weight?" My response was "a little."

In fact, I stayed mum about the whole thing! I figured that if my own family could be so unsupportive and skeptical, imagine what others would think and say to try to sabotage my success to date.

Subject: Question #5

Hey LA (not to be confused with the city),

First, I have a word-hack for you . . . h-e-double hockey sticks=HELL. I'm a big believer in keeping it real . . .

So your out-of-sight, out-of-mind strategy is one not enough people think of using. That's part of the systems approach I teach. Most of the ME problems we think we have are actually SYSTEM problems. Moving something out of sight is a very smart system approach.

I'm really glad you have addressed the whole family thing here. I get lots of questions on this and have little to offer being that I am a primal bachelor. Hey, I made up a new phrase. Maybe I should create a Being Primal Dating site? . . . or not

I'm very surprised teenaged kids would freak out about no treats in the house . . . ha ha!

Actually, I am more surprised when I see them eating something healthy. I am always tempted to walk up and slap it out of their hand and say, "What the hell is wrong with you. You're a teenager. Stop putting healthy food in your body."

To be honest, most adults act the same way . . . and as you said, it's surprising how sabotage-y (yes, I am making up words now) people can be.

BUT, that's a huge insight you made. People need to understand that many of those around them, because of their own fears and insecurities, will project their own problems on them. And we somehow feel we need to take ownership of those problems. WE DON'T!

Good for you for picking up on this when you first saw it.

I'm really intrigued by this, so question 5 is this . . .

I want to dig in a little deeper here. In this line here, you say,

Normally this type of conflict would have me settle back into our old way of doing things . . . but there was something different about this.

Expand on this for me. What strategies did you use to prevent this? Were you journaling? Did you have some sort of mantra? Were you thinking of putting the kids up for adoption? Let me in on the inner workings of what was different.

DD

Subject: Response to Question #5

Dean, you crack me up! And yes, h-e double hockey sticks, does equal HELL . . . I was just being creative.

To be honest, I can't really explain why this time was different. I can only say I felt rebellious, like I was undergoing some secret transformation, both physically and mentally.

It was as if ceasing to eat grains and sugar actually gave me mental clarity. I felt physically strong, and mentally I felt able, something that having been clinically depressed for years never allowed me to feel.

At first it was just about "outta sight, outta mind," but then came a family birthday party, which meant temptation and questions from observers.

I went; I nibbled and stayed within my dietary guidelines. When asked what I was doing to lose weight, I simply said, "It's all just eating healthy and exercising." The "new" selfish me wasn't about to give out this fabulous secret, but I also didn't want to be responsible for anyone else's body.

For example, as the weight and inches came off, my husband began to see that maybe there was something to this whole paleo/primal thing, so he began to reduce his bread intake and stopped drinking fruit juices. But he wasn't eating eggs or nearly enough protein, so I had to tell him to research what was right for HIS body. I didn't want something to go wrong and have him blame it on me and/or the diet. For me it was about going whole hog, not halfway, in order to see results, and I wasn't about to lead people on a path until I was sure it was good and safe.

The first three months I did keep a journal/record of my measurements, weight, and just little things I would notice about my moods, feelings, relationships, ability/inability to handle situations, bathroom habits, and foods that triggered a craving response, and this helped me immensely by keeping it all real for me. I started to talk to friends and close family members about what I was doing, but was met with so much negativity that I just stopped. I didn't want to spend my time trying to defend my choices . . . but I carried on.

At this point I had lost just over 25 pounds and needed to tell my doctor that I wanted off ALL my meds. So I made an appointment, but what he didn't know was that I had already stopped taking my meds two weeks before seeing him.

My weight was down, my blood pressure was normal, and he could tell my mental state was euphoric. He was happy and assumed that his 'low-fat' diet had finally kicked in. I didn't argue with him. I smiled and walked out of his office into the rain WITHOUT a stack of prescriptions to fill.

As for putting the kids up for adoption . . . the thought has crossed my mind many times over the years! Actually my kids are pretty awesome and quite proud of their mama . . . now!

Subject: Question #6

Hey Laurie Anne,

Yes, I do have my moments where those damn ducks finally agree to get into a row and my stuff actually comes out funny as intended. Unfortunately, I don't think people appreciate just how uncooperative (and selfish) ducks really are.

I love the brilliance of keeping a journal to record the things you recorded. People completely discount this, but as I said before,

"There are reasons why we do what we do (or don't do). If we fail to see that, we will never create lasting change because some recurring thought pattern from our past will rear its ugly head and derail our success as it has done to us consistently over the course of our lifetime."

So I'm jumping up to my fourth grade here, but am I right to assume that we are now into May 2011 and you have dropped 25 pounds and are completely medication free? (Oh, and wowzers about the med-free thing!)

If so, with question #6 I would like you to expand on this point you wrote by providing some specific examples . . .

The first three months I did keep a journal/record of my measurements, weight, and just little things I would notice about my moods, feelings, relationships, ability/inability to handle situations, bathroom habits, and foods that triggered a craving response, and this helped me immensely by keeping it all real for me.

I want to really get a clear picture of specific things you learned, and I would like you to share how you responded to some of these things.

DD

Subject: Response to Question #6

Dean,

Your ducks always seem to be lined up from what I can tell. I find your personality totally mesmerizing. I think you should have your own television show!

Keeping a journal was the only way to "talk" to someone about what I was doing without being judged and confronted. I wanted to be honest with myself, and this was the safest way for me.

I also did it, as I mentioned, to keep track of measurements, which were astounding! I wasn't losing tons of weight at first, but I was working out four times a week, a little cardio, but mostly weight training and body resistance exercises. The inches were coming off!

Below I've included my very first entry into my journal:

January, don't even care what day it is, 2011

BMI- waaaay to high to write down. (32.3 OBESE)

> *Weight-194lbs eeeekkkk!!!*
>
> *Waist-42.5 inches*
>
> *Chest-41.5 inches*
>
> *Under chest- 39 inches*
>
> *Hips-43 inches*

Great! I'm shaped like a freakin' barrel!!! *Sob*

I'm doing this! Nobody is stopping this freight train! I'm finally doing something for me! Bcuz I deserve it!

I can do this!

Some other entries along the way . . .

J. isn't being supportive, no big surprise there; he hates any kind of change. The problem is the kids are mirroring him...they are all sabotaging me.

I think they're all just jealous of my success. Or maybe I'm too sensitive...Nah, they're jealous!

My own Mom can't be supportive, she claims I must be starving myself...figures...not letting her get to me...ok maybe just a little bit. :(

OMG! I just realized that the more almond butter I eat the more I want...STAY AWAY FROM THE ALMOND BUTTER! Well...until further notice at least :)

Eating a tiny squeak of cheese seems to ward off craving for sweet crap. Good to know!

Bad night sleep=Cravings...F*%ck!! Shitty!

Must eat spinach every day! Good for regular bm's [bm=bowel movements]

BM's much smaller than before...no fillers *snicker*

July 25th, 2011

Sorry journal, I haven't been around much lately, been feeling a little too cocky and just winging it; been feeling great though! Even hubby has lost a few lbs and is all muscle...love it!

*Discovered some Paleo friendly treats to replace any temptations but they appear to be equally dangerous!! :(So I don't bake much anymore...my treat is now an iced coffee, literally brewed coffee over ice...or blueberries...or I buy myself a book/magazine or a new workout outfit (very motivating) I have noticed men staring!!! That hasn't happened since my 20's.... kinda makes my ego swell *giggle* I've still got it! Or rather...I just got it back! Yep! I've brought sexy back! :)*

Okay! Current stats:

>   *BMI- No clue! Don't care!*

>   *Weight-141 lbs*

>   *Waist-31.5 inches (damn thick waist!)*

>   *Under chest-33 inches*

>   *Chest-37.5inches*

>   *Hips-37inches*

Wish now I would have taken other measurements...legs, arms etc... Oh well, they all got smaller! Was wearing a size 16 and am now in a size 6!!!!!!!!!!!!!!!!!!!!!!!!!!!!

There you have it, a peek into my journal entries . . .

I will do another measurement/weigh in early September, but it seems that for now my body is at its comfort zone. My target goal is 135 pounds, but I'm not as worried about the numbers as I am about how I look and feel.

The journey continues . . .

Subject: Question #7

Hey Laurie Anne,

I loved the barrel comment, and I love the journal entries you have included. I think it is one of the best things people can do. It is amazing what we can learn, but more importantly it allows us to go back and get a glimpse at the "someone" we no longer are. (Wow! Is it just me or is that so deep I need to put up a warning sign!)

This is all about transparency. If people don't dive in and address their dirty details they will never make any lasting change.

I was particularly fascinated with the journal entries about the family members. We also learn a lot about other people when we embark on change. People's reactions are a reflection of their own fears. But most of us don't realize that we unknowingly take ownership of those and somehow feel we must prove them wrong.

That's a big problem for a lot of people. They are surrounded by people who struggle with anything that doesn't fit into their tiny view of how the world works.

Oh, and almond butter is also my nemesis. We do battle every few weeks. I always win, though, and demolish it within 24 hours. I'm considering a monthly relationship instead.

So before I talk to you more about your workouts, I wanted to address this whole family thing.

So question #7 is this . . .

Clearly, for reasons that had nothing to do with you, los familia unit was not supportive. How did you deal with that specifically? And has their stance softened now that you are no longer shaped like a barrel?

DD

PS . . . I love the fact you said you are no longer concerned so much about weight, but rather look. That outlook was HUGE for me in my transformation. I still have no idea how much I weigh, nor do I know how much I have lost.

Subject: Response to Question #7

Dean, I find it really interesting that you have no idea how much you weigh or have lost. At first I was obsessed with the scale! Then when I noticed that the clothing sizes went down, THAT was much more important, so now I weigh myself once a month, usually at the gym where they also figure out actual body fat percent and such. Good for you for not becoming a slave to the scale; it took me awhile to figure that one out.

My husband has definitely softened now that he can see and *ahem* feel . . . the results. It almost feels like our early courtship days when he couldn't take his eyes and hands off me. Too much information? Nah! Just tellin' it like it is!

He was constantly trying to sabotage my efforts by bringing home my favorite junk or just questioning my daily diet and whether I was getting enough of this or that. At the time it just frustrated me and made me angry. Now I realize he was just worried and being caring, but it was always about the approach. I felt that my entire world was being attacked. It still comes up occasionally, but now I just say, "You do what you do, and let me do what I do." That seems to do the trick.

He has even lost a few pounds himself by eliminating a lot of sugar and processed foods. I doubt he will ever go whole hog, but I am pleased that he is thinking twice about what he puts into his body and by going to the gym with me 4X's a week. He looks fabulous!

He still has problems with not being able to bring me home "treats" like he used to. He would pop into our favorite biscotti place, our favorite butter tart place, etc. once in a while to surprise me with a special treat. My barrel was living proof of my husband's adoration.

It has stopped. I have to keep reassuring him that his spending time with me is much more of a treat, or if he insists, I would love a magazine, a pint of blueberries, or some grass-fed butter. Also one aspect of spending time together is we can do many more outdoor activities. We go to the gym together; we take our road bikes out for a spin; we go on a hike together. . . . THOSE are the treats I want and need, not just for my health, but for the health of our marriage as well.

My children have stopped poking fun at me and are starting to just enjoy my mental clarity and ability to keep up with them. My son, 15, has made the attempt to go paleo a few times (so he can get a six pack), but says he can't give up eating junk. It doesn't fit in with his social life apparently.

My daughter has stopped eating bread, but still eats Pop Tarts and doughnuts. I don't talk them out of anything or into anything. If they ask, I explain.

The hardest family member to deal with was my mom. As I mentioned before, she would be a great candidate for this journey, and even though I invited her along, she wouldn't come. I'm not sure if she's proud of me, because she says things like, "You know it's unhealthy to starve yourself." Or, "You're going to make yourself sick if you don't eat. Are you eating?"

The best one came from a close friend "A woman your age shouldn't be so into vanity. You already have a husband." *sigh*.

Saying "No" to food is impossible at my parents'/in-laws'/friends' homes. "Just one bite." Or "It won't hurt you to try it."

At first it made me furious, and I would resist visiting anyone, but as time went by I realized that people just don't understand. My Mom is the person I'd most like to help, and she resists, but if I think about it I know exactly how she feels. I too felt trapped and had zero confidence to carry anything out. And just like me, she needs to have that moment . . . the moment when you realize, come hell or high water, you HAVE to do something to change the situation.

She needs to do that herself. . . . I can't force it onto her, just like nobody could have forced it on me. And so for now, I encourage, but mostly just smile, hug her, and tell her I love her.

I love my mom immensely, and I really hope she has her moment before it's too late for her health.

Hey Dean . . . maybe we should start a chapter of AA. . . Almond Butter Anonymous? I see you smiling . . . I know there must be others out there!

Subject: Question #8

Hey Laurie Anne,

That is correct. I have no idea how much I weigh or how much I have lost. Like you, I realized that a scale is horribly flawed. There are way too many intangibles that it does not measure, and quite frankly, many people end up sacrificing common sense (adopting calorie restriction for instance) and future sustainability to get immediate results NOW!

Unfortunately, that doesn't work, nor does it do anything for our self-esteem and confidence when we are a slave to those numbers on the scale.

So being primal (the lifestyle, not my site) has improved your marriage and strengthened your relationship with your kids. That's pretty dang amazing.

OK, so question number 8 then is this . . .

What is your exercise philosophy? And perhaps as you explain it you can wrap in examples of what a typical week of exercise might look like?

Also, I am curious to know how your routine has evolved since you started this 8 months ago and what changes you have seen in terms of the functionality of your body.

DD

PS . . . I don't think we need an association for our almond butter addiction . . . we just need to change the name. It's tough to resist anything with the name "butter" in it. Seriously, grind up rocks, put it in a jar and call it rock butter and I am all over it baby! If we change it to something like Almond Grease or Almond Manure, then it becomes much less glamorous.

Subject: Response to Question #8

I applaud you Dean for not being a slave to the scale; so many people out there on both sides of the coin, dieters and professionals who "help" them, become obsessed with the scale and lose sight of the things that really matter. In my opinion, being overly conscious of the numbers just leads to failure. If for some reason the scale rebels and the number lurches upward, it causes many to give up and deem themselves failures.

So this is the point in the interview where we get physical. I was looking forward to this! *wink*

Exercise for me was always a negative experience. I hated it as a young kid and into my teens. I was not interested in the least in sweating and burning calories. I preferred food, books, and music. In my adult years I have belonged to a couple of gyms . . . only to stop after a few weeks. Not to mention there was always a coffee house or great little bakery on the way to or from the gym . . . so I would go there instead. (Sad . . . I know.)

This time it's different. Seeing immediate body fat loss made me feel less embarrassed to go to the gym; I even bought myself a cute outfit, and my hubby bought me an iPod. I was armed and at least looked the part as I walked into the gym.

I met with a trainer, and he showed me some basic moves using my body as resistance, adding dumbbells for toning. It was a great place to start; the cardio stuff was easy! I did lunges ad nauseam . . . you should see my legs now!

Unfortunately, the next time I went in I felt alone and lost in a sea of hard-body men and women on the weight training floor, so I doubled my cardio that day instead. The next time I went in, there weren't a lot of people on the floor, so I did my thing. It felt great!

The next step for me was watching others and imitating them. I watched how they used the weights and machines and tried them out myself . . . but only when I was sure nobody was looking.

One day a lady came over to me looking exactly as I must have in the early days and asked me if I could help her figure out one of the machines. Then she asked if she was holding the weights correctly and with proper form. Huh? Did she mistake me for an employee? A professional trainer of sorts? I explained that I knew little, but was happy to share what I had learned.

Then it came to me. . . . I BELONGED!

That's the moment I became a gym rat. . . . Now don't get me wrong. I don't live at the gym, but I go three or four times a week.

I don't have a routine per se, but I like to shake things up; I may do a class one week, high-intensity interval training the next. Some days I will just do some laps in the lovely saltwater pool. One day a week is always my weight training day. And to be honest, I just go and lift heavy things until my arms are exhausted . . . and then I lift some more . . .

One day is always cardio. I shake it up with 10 minutes of treadmill running at 5–6 kilometers an hour on a 1 percent incline, then hit the elliptical for another 10 minutes and finish with the bike trainer for the last 10 minutes. Then I get down and into plank position and hold it for as long as possible, and then do 12 sit-ups, 12 push-ups, and work on my pull-ups . . . that's it!

The most important thing for me is that getting fit and feeling fabulous has also given me the confidence to open doors for myself. I recently bought a road bike so that I can now accompany my cycling devoted husband on long road rides, and we manage to go out at least once a week and ride anywhere from 12 to 18 km at a time.

At the cottage, I love taking the canoe out. Paddling is an awesome workout, not to mention the obvious hiking, swimming, and tree climbing!

So I guess my exercise philosophy would be to MOVE every day! The more you move, the more you will want to move. Trust me! Do things you love to do a lot! And try new things you've never tried before. I like to remind myself that the person you admire doing something was once a newbie as well.

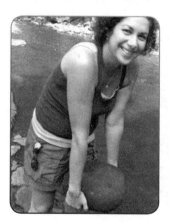 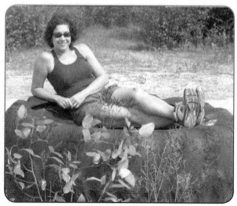

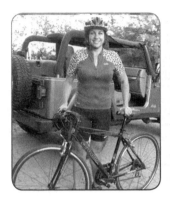
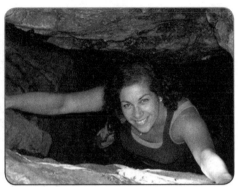

Subject: Question #9

Hey Laurie Anne,

You are so right on the number focus thing leading to failure. People focus on the number and completely forget that this is all about how we look and feel. Feeling great and loving how we look has nothing to with a number. If I had the power I would ban all scales.

I am so glad you shared the evolution of enjoying working out. You are bang on. It becomes easier to get into when we see fat loss happening. And it gets even more exciting once you start seeing muscle separation. I remember the first time I saw a slight separate in my shoulder. It was so motivating I actually cried. OK, I am kidding. I didn't cry, but damn it was exciting. Don't get me wrong. It was nothing anyone could see unless they were equipped with a magnifying glass, but I knew it was there, and workouts continued to get more intense as a result, and it seemed the results piled on fast.

And again the family theme comes back into play. I can't tell you how much I love that. I do think there is something about the primal/paleo movement that is very community driven. I just finished my interview with Sarah Fragoso as well, and I got the same sense from her. It has brought her and her family SO much closer together. It's really quite inspiring. So much so, I was going to ask her if she wanted to adopt a forty-five-year-old son, but then I realized she already had a three-year-old.

Great philosophy too! I love simplicity.

OK, so this takes me to question #9. What does a typical eating day look like for you? And what strategies or tips have you developed to help keep you on track? Oh, and what is your biggest temptation and how do you CRUSH IT!

DD

Subject: Response to Question #9

This is a copy of my early eating journal. As you can see I kept it pretty simple. Keeping it basic at first meant I didn't have to think about it.

These days I have opted to be a little more adventurous by:

- Eating fewer nuts and adding avocado instead. (I used to hate them!)

- I have also tried a few paleo/primal-friendly recipes for things like pancakes, just to vary from eggs.

- I will occasionally have a liquid breakfast if I am in a hurry, which is made up of frozen berries and spinach in a blender with some coconut milk and water. . . . Simple and good!

- I enjoy varying my veggies, and will have kale or other greens in place of spinach.

- I scour cookbooks (I collect them) for recipes I can tweak to be paleo-friendly. That way, even if I were having broccoli or cauliflower, it wouldn't taste or look the same every day.

- I make sure to drink plenty of water and green tea all day long, and will treat myself to the occasional brewed coffee over ice . . . yum!

- I have been enjoying eating our catch at the cottage; from lake to table is a fabulous thing!

- This fall I look forward to enjoying fresh deer up north with our local friends who hunt. As a former vegetarian . . . I would NEVER have dreamed of saying that!

- I eat a lot of meat, liver, fish, and eggs.

- I eat coconut oil by the spoonful occasionally, or just cook my veggies in it.

But even though it may appear that I've got it all under control . . . there are still triggers for me.

I am sure many people can identify with the chocolate obsession. I only eat Lindt 90 or 99 percent now, which is great! But the problem for me is it just makes me feel "snacky" for the rest of the day. The same happens with almond butter . . . I could probably eat the whole jar in one sitting! That $hit is good stuff!

So I proceed with caution. I do whatever it takes to distract myself from the craving. This usually involves leaving the house. I take the dog for a walk, go for a run, or go climb the monkey bars at the park.

If I still have the craving when I get back, then I take a square of chocolate, or a tablespoon full of almond butter (or sometimes both together) and indulge! It's OK! I am giving in to a craving, but I am making good choices. . . I am learning in this journey to replace my bad habits with good ones.

I will ALWAYS have cravings . . . PMS or otherwise. I have decided not to beat myself up over it, but to substitute my previous indulgences with healthy, more natural goodies.

Subject: Question #10

Hey Laurie Anne,

Your simplicity approach is brilliant. Decision making is draining and often sucks the life out of us. The fewer decisions we have to make (in all areas of our life), the more likely we are going to make the right decisions when we are required to make one.

The best way to sum up what you are doing is to say, for the most part, you have your eating on autopilot.

And thanks for clarifying the whole cravings thing.

That's another misconception out there. People think cravings disappear. They don't, but what happens over time is that voice inside our head goes from screaming, "I WANT THAT NOW!" to more of a whisper.

I'm so sad. This is the last of our ten questions.

So, I want you to play the role of teacher. There will be people reading this who will be inspired to give the paleo lifestyle a go.

Knowing what you now know, what are three things you would teach them to help ensure they have a successful experience? Use examples from your own life to back up your points as well.

DD

Subject: Response to Question #10

The last question . . . this makes me sad too, Dean! It's been such a great experience!

- So I could tell your readers about how much weight I've lost to date or
- What percent body fat I have lost or
- How many inches I have lost so far. . . .

But I remember reading those facts about other people and thinking, "Yeah right! It'll never work for me."

What impresses me is when people tell it like it is . . . the truth, the whole truth and nothing but!

> Tell me that it's OK to fall off the wagon sometimes as long as you dust yourself off and carry on the right path.

> Tell me that this is a journey, not a quick fix. Humans are waaaaay too complicated!

> Remind me that regardless of what my numbers are, I am #1 for taking on this lifestyle and bettering my health for the future.

If I had to stand up and tell anyone anything about this I would say:

First, ignore the naysayers. In fact, do this journey in stealth mode, just under the radar, until you can show them firsthand the changes going on in your body.

It was hard for me to deal with people's negativity until I had to buy new, smaller clothing and had the energy of a six-year-old. This gave me strength to show them without even having to justify what I was doing. In fact, the looks on their faces were priceless, and I didn't even have to say a word.

Second, I would remind everyone to keep it simple, especially at first. Keeping it simple means less stress! And simplicity will keep you from wondering if you're still on track. REMEMBER this is not a short-term diet. This is a lifestyle. You will never go back!

Keeping it simple, especially in the beginning, eliminated the need to figure out daily menus and whether or not I was eating the right amount of stuff. I figured out a menu that kept me full and I was seeing results, so I used it. Why fix what ain't broke . . . right?

When you get to your desired target (whatever that may be), you can play around with your food choices. Being creative is kinda like the next stage. Just when you begin to get bored, you step it up a notch! It's a lot of fun and there are so many great resources out there!

Sarah Fragoso's *Everyday Paleo* cookbook is my current favorite, and there are many other wonderful recipes out there.

Third, and probably most important, "listen to your body!"

During this journey, I have finally learned how to stop eating when I am full, even if I still have half the food on my plate.

As someone who would lick the plate clean and get seconds, this was a huge thing to learn. But on this eating plan I found it simple. My body told me when I was full.

Move! I can't stress enough how important it is to move! You don't need to have an expensive gym membership. You can walk your dog, go for a long walk in your neighborhood, walk to the store and bring shopping bags. Carrying heavy grocery bags is a great workout!

Ride your bicycle! It could be your new passion! Go to your nearest playground and be a kid again! I do this at least once a week. It's so much fun! Climb, hang, swing, and run.

Challenge someone to a friendly game of basketball, soccer, tennis, badminton . . . whatever you have access to. Your body will tell you when it needs to move. In fact, your body will constantly make you move.

BELIEVE me when I say I never thought in a million years that it would happen to me.

I will dance in the store to the music, use my kitchen counters to lift my body. I lift heavy rocks and tree trunks at the park . . . I climb trees . . .

So **Jump In**! You won't regret it!

For all those who stuck it through and read this interview . . . Thank You! It means a lot to me that you took the time.

Dean, this has been a great experience. You have made this yet another wonderful part of the journey for me.

Tell your tale

FROM WOE TO WOW! ✉

Tell me your story...

Here is a little reality check for you. Inspiring stories are great. But few of them lead to action if you aren't committed to a higher purpose.

You need to have a compelling vision connected to this transformation. If not, the moment the euphoria and newness of all the change wears off is also the moment you will begin to fall back on the self-defeating habits of your past.

My vision...

Not to go all Gandhi on you, but I think it is imperative to your success to commit to a higher purpose, to something greater than yourself.

Listen, I had no clue if I would be successful or not when I started, but one of the scenarios I did hitch my caboose to was a vision of teaching others how to transform their bodies.

The idea seemed insane at the time. Again, I had no idea if I would be successful or not, but I would have moments where I could see myself talking to hundreds of people at a seminar about the keys to creating sustainable transformation.

That was my secret little incentive that I had. I wanted to fix my own problem and then find a way to help others fix theirs.

And this book is a continuation of that vision! I have no doubt it wouldn't have happened had I not committed myself to a purpose greater than myself.

Story time...

So here is my way of helping you create purpose. I want to tell your success story. I want to use your transformation to inspire others to reclaim their bodies and their lives.

Make it your goal to have me tell your story. Not only will you drastically change your own life, but you will also have the opportunity to inspire thousands of others as they learn about your incredible tale.

So here are a few tips to get started.

1. Take a before picture of yourself (front view, side view, and back view).

2. Identify the shifts you are going to use.

3. Document the process: take notes of the insights you make.

4. Set a goal to tell me your story somewhere between four to six months from today.

5. Capture the journey via pictures and measurements.

6. **MAKE SHI**(F)**T HAPPEN!**

7. Send me your story!

8. Become an inspiration!

I wish you all the best and I can't wait to read your story.

To **MAKING SHI**(F)**T HAPPEN,**

Dean Dwyer

makeshifthappen.org
beingprimal.com

RESOURCES

Books about change...

- *Redirect: The Surprising New Science of Psychological Change,* Timothy D. Wilson

- *Mindset: The New Psychology of Success,* Carol Dweck

- *Linchpin: Are You Indispensible,* Seth Godin

- *Good To Great: Why Some Companies Make the Leap and Others Don't,* Jim Collins

- *The War of Art: Break Through the Blocks and Win Your Inner Creative Battles,* Steven Pressfield

- *Rework,* Jason Fried and David Heinemeier Hansson

- *Getting Real: The Smarter, Faster, Easier Way to Build a Successful Web Application,* Jason Fried and David Heinemeier Hansson

- *Switch: How to Change Things When Change is Hard,* Chip and Dan Heath

- *The Last Word on Power: Executive Re-invention for Leaders Who Must Make The Impossible Happen,* Tracy Goss

- *Influencers: The Power to Change Anything,* Kerry Patterson

- *Against the Odds: An Autobiography,* James Dyson

- *The Tipping Point: How Little Things Can Make a Big Difference,* Malcolm Gladwell

- *Mindless Eating: Why We Eat More Than We Think,* Brian Wansink

- *The Power of Less: The Fine Art of Limiting Yourself to the Essentials...in Business and in Life,* Leo Babauta

- *The Seven Habits of Highly Effective People: Powerful Lessons in Personal Change,* Steven Covey

- *The 4-Hour Body,* Tim Ferris

- *Banker to the Poor: Micro-lending and the Battle Against World Poverty,* Muhammad Yunus

Paleo Related Books...

- *The Paleo Solution: The Original Human Diet,* Robb Wolf

- *Everyday Paleo,* Sarah Fragoso

- *The Primal Blueprint: Reprogram Your Genes for Effortless Weight Loss, Vibrant Health and Boundless Energy,* Mark Sisson

- *The Paleo Diet: Lose Weight and Get Healthy by Eating the Foods You Were Designed to Eat,* Loren Cordain

- *Good Calories Bad Calories: Fats, Carbs and the Controversial Science of Diet and Health,* Gary Taubes

- *Paleo Comfort Foods: Homestyle Cooking for a Gluten-Free Kitchen,* Julie Sullivan Mayfield and Charles Mayfield

- *Make it Paleo: Over 200 Grain-Free Recipes For Any Occasion,* Bill Staley and Hayley Mason

- *Well Fed: Paleo Recipes for People Who Love to Eat,* Melissa Joulwan

- *Practical Paleo: A Customized Approach to Health and a Whole Foods Lifestyle,* Diane Sanfilippo

- *Eat like a Dinosaur: Recipe and Guidebook for Gluten-free Kids,* The Paleo Parents

- *Death by Food Pyramid,* Denise Minger

- *Primal Body, Primal Mind: Beyond the Paleo Diet for Total Health and a Longer Life,* Nora Gedgaudas

BLOGS...

Paleo Related...

- Mark's Daily Apple by Mark Sisson [www.markdailyapple.com]
- Robb Wolf [www.robbwolf.com]
- Free the Animal by Richard Nikoley [www.freetheanimal.com]
- Everyday Paleo by Sarah Fragoso [www.everydaypaleo.com]
- Fat Burning Man by Abel James [www.fatburningman.com]
- Paleo Lifestyle Diet by Sabastien Noel [www.paleodietlifestyle.com.com]
- Paleo Magazine [www.paleomagonline.com]
- Balanced Bites by Diane Sanfilippo [www.balancedbites.com]
- Cave Girl Eats by Liz Wolfe [www.cavegirleats.com]
- Chris Kresser [www.chriskresser.com]
- Underground Wellness by Sean Croxton [www.undergroundwellness.com]
- Living an Optimized Life by Dr Jack Kruse MD, Neurosurgeon [www.jackkruse.com]
- Primal Palate by Bill Staley and Hayley Mason [www.primal-palate.com]
- Paleo Comfort Foods by Julie and Charles Mayfield [www.paleocomfortfoods.com]
- Whole 9 Life by Melissa and Dallas Hartwig [wwwwhole9life.com]
- Nom Nom Paleo [www.nomnompaleo.com]
- Nerd Fitness by Steve Kamb [www.nerdfitness.com]
- The Bulletproof Executive by Dave Asprey [www.bulletproofexecutive.com]
- Primal Toad by Todd Dosenberry

[www.primaltoad.com]

- Civilized Caveman Cooking Creations by George Bryant [www.civilizedcavemancooking.com]
- The Clothes Make the Girl by Melissa Joulwan [www.theclothesmakethegirl.com]
- Raw Food SOS by Denise Minger [www.rawfoodsos.com]
- Ancestral Health Society [www.ancestryfoundation.com]
- Paleo FX [www.paleofx.com]
- Efficient Exercise by Keith Norris [www.efficientexercise.com
- Primal Wellness Today [www.primalwellnesstoday.com]

Non-Paleo Lifestyle...

- The Art of Non-Conformity by Chris Guillebeau [www.chrisguillebeau.com]
- Zen Habits by Leo Babauta [www.zenhabits.net]
- Smart Passive Income by Pat Flynn [www.smartpassiveincome.com]
- Seth's Blog by Seth Godin [www.sethgodin.typepad.com]
- In Over Your Head with Julien Smith [www.inoveryourhead.net]
- TED [www.ted.com]
- Getting Stronger by Todd Becker [www.gettingstronger.org]

Podcasts...[search these in iTunes]

- Balanced Bites with Liz Wolfe and Diane Sanfilippo
- The Paleo Solution with Robb Wolf
- Livin' La Vida Low Carb Show with Jimmy Moore
- Everyday Paleo with Sarah Fragoso

- Latest in Paleo with Angelo Coppola
- Underground Wellness with Sean Croxton
- Revolution Health Radio with Chris Kresser
- Fat Burning Man with Abel James
- Bulletproof Executive with Dave Asprey and Armi Legge

You Tube Channels...

- Six Pack Shortcuts
- Body Rock TV
- Yogatic
- Underground Wellness
- Ross Training